C000096626

THE SEVEN KEYS TO STRENGTH TRAINING FOR MEN OVER 50

LEARN EVERYTHING YOU NEED TO LOSE FAT AND
GAIN MUSCLE, EVEN AS A COMPLETE BEGINNER

BRYANT WILLIS

© **Copyright 2021 - All rights reserved.**

The content contained within this book may not be reproduced, duplicated or transmitted without direct written permission from the author or the publisher.

Under no circumstances will any blame or legal responsibility be held against the publisher, or author, for any damages, reparation, or monetary loss due to the information contained within this book, either directly or indirectly.

Legal Notice:

This book is copyright protected. It is only for personal use. You cannot amend, distribute, sell, use, quote or paraphrase any part, or the content within this book, without the consent of the author or publisher.

Disclaimer Notice:

Please note the information contained within this document is for educational and entertainment purposes only. All effort has been executed to present accurate, up to date, reliable, complete information. No warranties of any kind are declared or implied. Readers acknowledge that the author is not engaged in the rendering of legal, financial, medical or professional advice. The content within this book has been derived from various sources. Please consult a licensed professional before attempting any techniques outlined in this book.

By reading this document, the reader agrees that under no circumstances is the author responsible for any losses, direct or indirect, that are incurred as a result of the use of the information contained within this document, including, but not limited to, errors, omissions, or inaccuracies.

CONTENTS

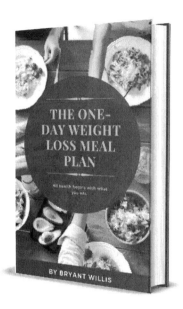

Before we get acquainted, I'd like to tell you about a concise book I made to complement what you're about to read. The cornerstone of supreme fitness is a healthy diet. That is why I have devised a meal plan to help you lose fat and sustain a happy body.

However, I thought that pushing a sale after you just bought one of my books would be unfair and a little greedy. So, instead, I've decided to give you this one for free!

Here is a little sneak preview of what value you will be getting out of this free book:

- An entire day of delicious meals laid out for you, designed specifically to help you lose fat
- Alternative meals to mix things up so you will never get bored
- Vital information on what foods to eat and ones to stay away from so you can become an expert on weight loss

As I said, it's free, so you might as well take a look inside. It's a very straightforward process. All you have to do is type bryantjwillis.com into your internet search bar and you will be taken to a page asking for your email address. This is so I can send you The One Day Weight Loss Meal Plan.

bryantjwillis.com

I hope you love it!

THE BEGINNING OF A JOURNEY

We all age. Some will approach this process gracefully, and some may try to cling to youth for as long as they can, but no matter how we feel, aging is inevitable, and it will happen to everyone. It is an undeniable truth of the world we live in. Moreover, with aging comes a set of consequences that we must deal with:

Our muscle mass grows more and more depleted with each day.

- Our bones grow weaker.
- The body experiences a natural loss of testosterone which is a factor in many other things.

I am a strong advocate of being proud of who you are and being comfortable with yourself, but that doesn't mean you have to roll over and accept your fate. We carve our own paths in life, and the process of aging cannot even come close to stopping that. All it takes is the ability to put your effort in to counteract these laws of nature. I am here to help you fight back and take control of your life.

I once had a friend, Clara, who was in her 30s. She had just gotten married to a man named James, a widower, who had two kids from his late wife, and was in his early 50s. James and Clara had fallen in love at first sight when they met at one of my friend's parties. Although there were over 15 years between them, you could tell they had a real connection. It was obvious. They began dating and decided to further their love life by getting married. Before their marriage, they started having problems in the bedroom, with James stating he wasn't "in the mood." My friend Clara is a charming and patient person, so she waited for him in hopes of this phase passing. A few months went past into their dry marriage. Clara, in desperation, began contemplating seeing her ex again (this was a guy who maltreated her), not for any reason other than sex. James couldn't satisfy her sexually. He had taken a look in the mirror and didn't like what he saw. He felt inadequate in bed because he was acutely aware of the age gap and its effects on his body. He thought this made him unattractive to Clara, this was not how Clara felt, but these thoughts had already sunk their claws deep into James's mind.

A fatal miscommunication as Clara assumed it was his loss of lust for her. What she couldn't get in James, she sought once more in Dan, her ex. We got talking one day, and she opened up to me about her dilemma. I understood the situation well, "A straightforward problem to solve," I told her. I asked for her permission to intervene. I got close to James, invited him to some of my workout sessions, got him involved in regular training. Over time James's attitude shifted; he grew confident enough to look himself in the mirror and be proud of the man he saw looking back at him. This confidence transitioned smoothly into a great sexual relationship with his partner. He could now express to Clara his previous concerns about his body because they no longer had a hold of his life. Today, their relationship is stronger than ever.

Recalling this incidence gives me a plethora of emotions. Although everything worked out in the end, that problem could have been the end of their marriage. Utterly unknown to him, James suffered from low levels of testosterone which affected his sexual drive and his ability to have satisfying sex. Regular exercise can raise testosterone levels because it increases muscle mass. The increase in muscle mass can lead to more testosterone in the body. Testosterone and many other aspects are why it is so essential to practice strength training as you get older, and this is why it is my dream to get you there.

There are so many men out there like James battling the loss of muscle mass as they age, a buildup of fat, and loss of strength, making the discharge of their daily activities challenging. It can be highly frustrating when your lack of fitness prevents you from doing things you used to do effortlessly. Unfortunately, some think their age restricts them from losing fat or gaining muscles; they believe they are too old to start exercising. Factually, regardless of your age, you need to stay fit, and I would go so far as to say it's way more important in the later years of your life than ever before.

You are not too old to hit the gym. No matter your age, you need to stay fit at all times because it is imperative to your mental and physical health. The older you get, the more challenging it becomes for you to deal with daily activities, and it gets worse when you do not have a lifestyle of fitness. There are some misconceptions about the types of fitness exercises that people between 50 and 70 can get involved in. According to the design of our bodies, as you get older, fitness may not be concentrated on long hours of training to chisel the abs out. Instead, the workouts I teach focus on helping you stay fit and mitigating the risks of suffering cardiovascular diseases. While still building muscle mass and increasing your balance. When you get to 50 and above, it is vital to cognizance your health, strength, and fitness.

Countless health issues arise from not exercising or not taking exercise seriously. These issues become more complicated as we age. Muscles may become stiffened from lack of exercise and lead to pain and uneasiness in movements. However, After reading all of this, I do not want you to get disheartened and despair over your age, lack of exercise, and inconsistent exercise lifestyle. It's never too late. You can be healthy, fit, and get that incredible body you never had, even as a young man!

Now I ask that you do a favor for me. Please make a conscious decision to take action on this book and give yourself the determination to live a healthy lifestyle. Worry less about the chances of getting injured, the information in this book will provide you with everything you need to train in the safest way possible so you can say goodbye to injures. You have most of the motivation you need in this book, but the rest needs to come from you! After going through each chapter (if you follow my advice), you should be on your way to becoming that fit, healthy man everyone marvels at. Fortunately, you do not have to do it alone. This book will take you through the seven most important things you need to achieve your dream body. By the end of this book, I am confident you will have learned a ton of information you can apply to your life, and I will have gained your trust.

If you are new to fitness and strength training, you have made the right decision by investing in this book. I have been in the fitness business as an instructor for just over ten years. It is my passion to help you achieve all of your body goals. Let me first clarify to you it does not have to be strenuous, and you do not need to spend long hours at the gym; you only need to be determined enough to push through the challenging parts. I want to help you get it right, and that is why I have put this book together. Through years of experience, I have garnered knowledge about fitness in general and, more specifically, men's fitness between the ages of 40 and above. I know how great the benefits are to training your body and positively changing your life.

Okay, now that you know a bit of me and what I am offering you, I hope you understand the value of this book. So, without further ado, let's jump right into it!

UNDERSTANDING THE POWER OF STRENGTH TRAINING PAST 50

One belief you could harm yourself with is to think you missed your chance, so there is no point in starting. Wrong. Opportunities will always present themselves to you. It's never too late for you to pick up a practice, change or work on improving a negative attitude, start a venture or profession, and many more.

Do you know Dwight Muhammad Qawi? Despite starting his career at an old age in boxing terms, Dwight enjoyed a great career at the top of the heap. Dwight finally got involved in the sport at the very late age of 25. To make matters worse, his journey started while serving time in Rahway State Prison for armed robbery. As you can imagine, this man was at an all-time low in his life. Most people wouldn't expect him to ever amount to anything. But there will always be a way out of the darkness, no matter what. He crawled out of the depths of despair and later on captured world titles in two weight classes, light-heavyweight, and cruiserweight. Tim Thomas, Randy Johnson, Didier Drogba, Antonio Gates, Bill Durnan, Hakeem Olajuwon, Kurt Warner are all athletes who started late in their various fields and still went on to make their mark on the sands of time. There are tens of thousands more.

What is Strength Training

As I would define it, strength training is any physical activity designed to increase muscle mass or fitness in a specific muscle group - an exercise using a resistant force to add stress to the engaged muscles.

It involves indulging your muscles more than its usual work rate. You overload your muscles. Any exercise can count as strength training if it consists of a medium to high-level effort and works on primary muscle groups in the body. You should know that strength training is not just about lifting weights in a gym to build your body. It goes a lot deeper than that.

We can divide older strength trainees into three categories: those who never stopped training, those who relapsed, and those who never trained at all. But the benefits of strength training as you grow beyond 50 are undeniable. Strength training is a significant part of the body's overall fitness that has lots of benefits to everyone, primarily those with health issues such as obesity, high or low blood sugar levels, heart disease, arthritis, and many more. Studies have shown that strength training can counteract muscle weakness and physical frailness in older people.

Types of Strength Training

There are several types of strength training: isometric strength training, isotonic strength training, and isokinetic strength training. Don't worry if you're still wondering what any of this means. I will explain.

Isometric Strength Training: It is also known as static strength training. This type of exercise recruits muscles and exert tension without really lengthening or shortening the muscles. Your muscles are flexed but not expanding or compressing. Isometric training often involves moves that target your whole body. And it's perfectly acceptable if you perform activities that can engage your entire body all at once. Isometric exercises are well suited for those with limited workout space, knee discomfort, or if you need a change in your typical fitness routine. Examples of isometric exercise are plank and side bridge, wall sit, and many yoga poses such as chair and tree poses. However, since these moves improve strength in one body position, they should complement more dynamic exercise regimens.

Isotonic Strength Training: Isotonic training keeps the muscle at the same tension or tone while it gets shortened. Many exercises you can think of are isotonic. You are moving your body out against an external weight or force through a range of motion intentionally. You are most likely familiar with most of the isotonic exercise regimen: squats, pull-ups, push-ups, stairs climbing, deadlifts, etc.

Isokinetic Strength Training: Isokinetic training makes you constantly work at a range of motion. Most isokinetic exercise uses specialized exercise machines that produce a continuous force regardless of how much effort you expend. The device controls the pace of the activity by fluctuating resistance throughout your set range of motion. Your speed or movement remains constant regardless of how much effort you exert. The speed and range of motion can be set to a target to suit your needs. Isokinetic exercise can test and improve your muscular strength and endurance. Using the stationary cycle, which you can find at your local gym for a workout, is a perfect example of isokinetic training.

The Testosterone Factor

Most men over 50 seem to experience an inevitable loss of strength, energy, and vigor. But it shouldn't be so. The frailness and reduced energy we often associate with aging include difficulty walking for long distances, climbing, and carrying loads. And these are all primarily due to muscle loss. The fact is, one of the main factors causing this muscle loss is inactivity. Let me give you a hypothetical example: pitch two men in their mid-50s, one man who has had years of training and being active with his body, and the other who spends most of his time sitting in front of the television watching old movies. Let's say you asked them to perform the same task, one they have never done before, but it involves physical strain and a small amount of flexibility. Who are you betting performs that task better? The one who has always been invested in strength training will do better. And with ease. This scenario might seem obvious to you but let's dissect this a bit. Firstly, the task is not strange to his body, and it has already grown a custom to doing kind of movements; secondly, his endurance is much higher, meaning his body is well equipped to deal with the strain. In this regard, that old saying is true for muscles: you either use them or lose them. Constantly engaging your muscles will help you with doing any physical tasks. And strength training is by far one of the best ways to develop those muscles.

All men naturally suffer a drop in testosterone as we age. According to a report by David Paolone, a urologist at UW Health's Men's Health Clinic, "Nearly 39 percent of men ages 45 years and older have low testosterone. A low level is considered below 300 nanograms per deciliter. And the prevalence of low testosterone grows with age: estimates show that it affects 12 percent of men in their 50s, 19 percent in their 60s, 28 percent in their 70s, and 49 percent in their 80s" (UW Health, 2017).

For those wondering what the hell testosterone is, let me explain. It's a hormone found in humans and other animals. It is the crucial male sex hormone (also found in females but with a much lower concentration). In men, testicles are the primary producers of testosterone. It regulates sex drive and plays a vital role in sperm production, fertility, muscle mass, bone density, fat distribution, and red blood cell production. I hope now you can see the importance of this hormone. Production of testosterone increases during puberty and starts to drop after age 30. after you pass 30, the testosterone level in men starts to slowly drop at a rate of around 1 percent per year on average. The drop in testosterone level is a natural result of aging. Testosterone affects so many functions. It can lead to hypogonadism (a condition where the body doesn't produce enough male hormones or sperm) or infertility when it drops below a certain level that is considered healthy. Another significant effect of low testosterone is the loss of muscle mass.

Testosterone plays a huge role in the development and regulation of muscle mass, and reduced hormone levels can result in a significant loss of muscle. Although low testosterone causes a drop in mass, the function and strength of the muscles do not diminish. Muscle mass is simply the muscle in your body, including the skeletal muscles, smooth muscles, and cardiac muscles. Low muscle mass has its associated health risks. It can negatively impact your overall health.

"Low muscle mass is associated with outcomes such as higher surgical and post-operative complications, a longer length of hospital stay, lower physical function, poorer quality of life and shorter survival."

— WITHINGS, 2021

Benefits of Strength Training

Many men think strength training is just for building biceps and an elusive six-pack. Perhaps that's one reason older men won't consider it. They don't care much about how their body looks and how others perceive them. I want to state that this way of living is entirely acceptable, but strength training is beyond that. If you're going to build bigger biceps, strength training is essential for making that happen. However, even if maxing out your muscle size isn't your objective, strength training is still one of the best ways to reach your health goals. Before your next workout, let me take you through some of the benefits of strength training, so you would take your exercise and subsequent sessions with the knowledge of why you put your body through it.

Strength and Fitness.

This is quite obvious, yet we can't overlook it. Strength training makes you stronger and fitter. Muscle strength is fundamental to carry out tasks daily, more so as you get into your 50s and naturally start to lose muscle mass. Strength training lowers the risk of having difficulty executing daily activities due to a lack of muscular fitness. These daily activities might include climbing up and down a set of stairs, moving furniture or other heavy objects, engaging in sporting activities or hiking, and even just standing for long periods. In short, it takes the fun out of the things you love to do when you're not fit and are unable to do them to the best of your ability.

Protection of Bone Health and Muscle Mass.

Once we clock 30 or thereabout, we start losing an average of 1% of lean muscle mass every year, as stated earlier. According to a study published in 2017 for Bone and Mineral Research, it was found that functional performance was improved through 30 minutes twice a week of high-intensity resistance and impact training. They also recorded higher bone density, structure, and strength in postmenopausal women with low bone mass, with no adverse effects (Watson, Weeks, Weis, Harding, Horan, Beck, 2017). Also, it is noted in the HHS guidelines that, for everyone, strength training activities help preserve or increase muscle mass which is vital for bone, joint, and muscle health as we age (U.S. Department of Health and Human Services, 2018).

Regulates Excess Weight

Many people think losing fat is about burning off as many calories as you can, so this might deter them from strength training because it's not focused on achieving this. There are many more forms of exercise that prioritize this. For example, aerobic exercise such as walking, running, swimming helps you increase the number of calories you burn off your body; this can 100% help you to shred some pounds. But strength training is also helpful even if you're not burning so many calories during your workouts. Many research affirms that strength training is beneficial for weight loss because it helps increase your resting metabolism. When you have a good strength training workout, it increases your excess post-exercise oxygen consumption. Your body continues to burn out calories after a strength training workout. Strength training keeps your metabolism active after the workout, much more than after aerobic activity. A study published about "Obesity" in 2017 documented three sets of dieters: dieters who didn't exercise, those who did only aerobic exercise, and dieters who performed strength training exercises four times a week for 18 months. Dieters who did strength training lost the most fat, averaging 18 pounds. Compared to the aerobic exercisers who lost 16 pounds and the dieters who didn't exercise only losing 10 pounds!

Development of Better Body Mechanics

Your body becomes more balanced, coordinated, and well postured. Older people are at a higher risk of falling because of inadequate physical functioning. You can reduce the risk of falling by some pretty high margins through a strength training exercise. Body balance is dependent on the strength of the muscles that keep you on your feet. The stronger your muscles, the better and steadier the balance.

Osteoporosis Prevention and Management

Osteoporosis is a health condition commonly found in older people. The condition weakens the bones, making them more likely to break. It can develop over several years, so people don't realize it's happening most of the time.

Muscular bodies have strong bones. Strength training significantly increases your bone mineral density. Any weight-bearing exercise that involves gravity pulling down on your body stresses you and helps strengthen the bones and muscles. Also, every time a muscle contracts, it pulls on the bone attached to it, which arouses the cell in the bone to secrete structural proteins that move minerals into the bone. If you want great results in this regard, focus on standing weight-bearing, such as squats and lunges. In a 2014 Journal of Family and Community Medicine study, just 12 weeks of strength training with squats increased lower spine and femur (thigh) bone mineral density by 2.9 and 4.9 percent, respectively.

Management of Chronic Diseases

Many studies have documented the numerous benefits of strength training to help other health issues. Strength training has been shown to help people in managing chronic diseases. If you have arthritis, strength training can be as effective as medication in decreasing arthritis pain. Or you have low or high blood sugar strength training can help stabilize your blood sugar levels and improve the use of insulin in your body.

Boosting of Energy Levels and Improvement of Moods

When you engage in strength training, your level of endorphins gets elevated, which, in turn, lift energy levels and improve your mood. All exercises boost your mood and give you a sense of happiness. Still, for strength training, additional research that's looked at our body's responses to such workouts offers further evidence that supports it has a positive effect on the brain (Strickland and Smith, 2014). Also, there is evidence showing strength training may help you sleep better.

Burning of More Calories: Your metabolism is boosted. Strength training helps boost the calories you burn during and after your workout. When you perform strength training, your body demands more energy based on how much you're exerting (meaning the intenser you're working, the more energy is required). after the workout, your body goes into a state of recovery which burns even more calories because it needs the energy to heal.

Cardiovascular Health Benefits

Along with aerobic exercise, muscle-strengthening physical activity helps improve blood pressure. I recommend you doing muscle-strengthening activities twice a week plus 150 minutes of moderately intense workouts at minimum to help reduce hypertension and minimize the risk of heart diseases.

Longer Lifespan:

Perhaps one of the most valuable benefits of strength training is the probability that it will lead to a longer life. A 2015 study in The Lancet found that grip strength accurately predicts death from any cause. The study suggests that lean muscle mass better measures a person's overall health. Having solid muscles has a direct correlation to living a longer life.

Getting Started with Strength Training

Maybe you are completely new to strength training, perhaps you have experience and are well versed in training your body, but you're looking for a better routine. You might be somewhere in between but find it hard to stay consistent. Whatever the case, let's start your training afresh, a clean slate from now on. Let me guide you through everything, and if you follow my plan right down to every detail, I guarantee you this journey will be a breeze. First, you need to commit. It's easy to start something, but to persevere through thick and thin, takes genuine skill. You have to be sure of the benefits you stand to achieve and beyond that, making it a lifelong attitude. There is no need to be intimidated by this because once you learn it and adapt it to your life, it becomes easy, and you will find yourself enjoying every moment of it.

Strength training comes down to two simple things:

- The movement of any weight against a resisting force. It can even be your body weight. Any exercise that puts high stress on your muscles can be considered strength training.
- Progressive overloading, doing more than the last time. Let's say you started with five push-ups today; in 1 week, you're doing 6. Your muscles will have to constantly adapt and rebuild to get stronger.

Knowing these principles is the foundation of your strength training journey.

.

1

THE FIRST KEY
A MENTAL FORTRESS

What is attitude? How do you explain it in tangible terms to understand it perfectly? In psychology, an attitude refers to beliefs, emotions, and behaviors toward a particular person, object, thing, or situation. Simply put, attitude is an inward feeling that impacts or is responsible for the way we act.

I once gave an illustration to my friend while teaching him about attitude some years ago to inform him how mindset affects our actions. I asked him what he would do if he were driving and got hit by another vehicle. Bear in mind that nobody was injured, and there was very little damage to the car. After a bit of back and forth trying to understand the hypothetical situation, he agreed that the offender would have to pay for the damages one way or another - an appropriate response. Then I asked what he would do if the offender got out of his vehicle, and it turned out to be me… this sparked a much different response, a kinder reaction that I must say I was a little flattered by. We agreed that he might let me off or accept minimal compensation because he knew me, and there weren't any noticeable damages to their car. Then I asked them the difference between a random offender and me; after all, we are both humans. The difference was they know me. They have a certain mindset (inward feeling) towards me. The attitude you have changes how you deal with the situation, which changes the outcome.

Our mindset is critical in everything we do, and you will need the right attitude if you are going to make strength training a part of your lifestyle. You need to know why you chose to pursue this goal and how to keep it up. Phycologist James Allen stated, "a person cannot travel within and stand still without." The same is true that a person cannot be stagnant within and travel outside. This may sound confusing at first so let me reiterate it another way. You cannot hope to achieve much in life if you are not prepared to change your mind. It would be best to work on your "inward feeling." first. Then with time, the outward actions match the inward thoughts.

Let me help you build the right attitude and develop a positive mindset towards your strength training success.

Why do you want to train? I find this imperative to ask, "Why do you wanna train?" you should ask yourself this question; I believe you will be more sincere with yourself, "why am I doing this?". This simple question is essential and should be asked by you every time you embark on something new.

You need to know why you want to train. This question is your motivating factor, your first and immediate fuel for the lifelong journey ahead. It's one factor that will always help you when you get tired and want to quit. There's a saying, "anytime you think of quitting, remember why you started in the first place." If you started without a solid reason, then quitting becomes inevitable when you encounter the slightest challenges in your journey.

That reminds me of a girlfriend I had during my years at high school. She was a pretty girl, but she ate a lot of shit (sorry for the language, but it's true). She was in good shape at the time, but I wanted to help her maintain that health because I knew she was headed in the wrong direction. So I pleaded and pleaded for her to come to the gym with me and try it out. After a lot of convincing, she decided to give it a go just to shut me up. I would be lying if I said our relationship was perfect, and over time, I realized That good looks in a girl is meaningless when that girl makes you miserable. As you can probably guess, we broke up after five months of being together. The irony of the story is I never saw her in that gym again. And yes, that might have been due to her not wanting to deal with us meeting in the hallways and those awkward encounters, but I genuinely think it was because she lacked conviction. Her reasons for going were centered around what I wanted, and when I was out of the picture, she had none.

You need to be personally convinced to train: Okay, so now you might be wondering to yourself, what's the best reason to train? The truth is there isn't one. Everyone is motivated by different things because we are all unique. Several factors can fuel your conviction. It might be one of the benefits that we covered in chapter one. It might be a way for you to escape life and invest your time in something meaningful. It might even be as simple as you want that toned 6 pack to use as a pleasant surprise for any girls you meet. Anything that will fuel your conviction, make sure it's something for you and not just a way to stop someone from moaning. Once your mind is made up, my friend, we're good to go. Let's roll on...

Your conviction births self-motivation that you need to launch yourself out into something new. Don't worry if you start this journey, and it's a little hard to make that commitment every day. There is a nice little trick your brain uses on you when you perform something enough times; it goes like this: you want to do something pretty challenging; you start with the bit of motivation you have only to find out the more you do it the easier it gets. The consistency of doing the same task builds a little section in your brain that lets you know it's that time again. And the best part is, your brain will reward you with Dopamine, also known as the "feel-good" hormone, every time you finish that task.

Create time to train: Strength training coach Bobby Maximus said, "Much of the training discussion focuses on training and nutrition, but one of the biggest obstacles people have when it comes to training is finding enough time. Time management seems to be the biggest determinant in a person's success in any given training program."

I don't want to assume you have plenty of time or that you don't have any time at all. In all honesty, it doesn't matter. When I think about time, I think of this saying, "if you want to do something, you'll find a way; otherwise, you find an excuse." Also, if it's important to you, I believe you'll create time for it. Having gone through the benefits of training and decided why you want to do this, it now comes down to making time even out of thin air if we have to. Bobby Maximus went on to say, "I've trained many different types of people with varying commitment levels. On average, I am disappointed with the amount of time people are willing to commit. So, I want to make one thing clear: time is not an excuse. The real issue is usually that a person isn't dedicated enough or has poor time management skills".

If it's time management that's standing in your way, then let me help you with it. We all have 24 hours for each day. How we use this time is entirely left to us. If you can manage your time very well, you can easily carve out about three hours every week for your training and be consistent with it. Use this guide I've made down below to manage your priorities, and you'll discover the extra time you never thought you had:

- High Importance / High Urgency: These come first above everything else.
- High Importance / Low Urgency: You can set deadlines to complete these projects or get these projects and fit them into your day, doing small amounts at a time.
- Low Importance / High Urgency: You should find quick, efficient ways to get this work done without much personal involvement. Plan these out ahead of time so you can them out of the way as soon as possible.
- Low Importance / Low Urgency: These are tedious or repetitious tasks, such as a filling. Stack them up and do all of it together once every week, or get somebody else to do them, or don't do them at all.

Plan out your week with this in mind to maximize your work efficiency.

Set goals when starting: What is velocity? Simple: velocity is speed plus direction. Make sure you understand the difference between velocity and speed. Speed alone is useless when you have no focus. Setting out on a strength training program without a goal is the same. You must set goals, figure out what you aim to achieve. Without goals, you cannot measure progress, and you can get tired and weary along the way at any point. Also, if you have clear milestones in place, it will boost motivation every time you pass one of those milestones. One of the best motivators is proven success, so use that to your advantage.

Get social support

Many people overlook and underestimate the use of social support. Social support from fellow men going through a strength training program can be a big jackpot for beginners and even experienced trainees looking for people to share their success with. Having like-minded people around you makes it much easier to convey emotions, questions, struggles, and achievements. With the support of others in a similar position to your own, you will not fail or deflate because the group won't let you!

There are many ways to join a group, but approaching people in person can be a little intimidating. A great way to get around this is to become a part of a community through social media. My recommendation is Facebook. Here you can find millions of groups worldwide and hundreds that share the same goals as you. It's simple to join them; all you have to do is go into the search bar and type in what you're looking for. You might not be a social media type of guy, so another great way is to register at a gym; you can connect with other men above 50 for social support. The struggles of others will let you that you're not alone.

On the other hand, their success stories will serve as sources of inspiration and let you know your goal of adopting a strength training program is achievable. It will clear up your mind about any doubt you might have concerning strength training. I urge you not to underestimate the importance of friendship.

Also, you could complete training together with a group or even have friendly competitions to stir and inspire passion amongst the group. Studies have shown that friendly matches help individuals to try harder. It certainly applies to me. I have been told by friends that I can sometimes get a bit too competitive (especially in board games).

When the doubt kicks in: You might get weary along the line, that's the truth. You might find yourself getting tired with all the hard work or not getting the desired results. When you feel you are not getting the desired results, quitting (although easy) is the worst option. Take a pause, review your program, make sure it's not a case of you expecting so much in the space of little time or you expecting a result totally out of the box. This false judgment is common among people, but I want you to understand that life is a marathon, not a sprint. You need to prepare for the long hall and take it all in strides. If you're experiencing pain, you might need to reduce whatever weight you're training with or reduce the number of repetitions or sets. It's better to move slowly and steadily than hastily and burn out fast.

Don't compare yourself with others: There is a saying, "comparison is a thief of joy." You might find yourself in a similar situation to the following: You have been going about your workout plan faithfully and seeing results along the way, which makes you feel good, but you run into your friend who started around the same time as you and saw he had made more progress, then, you begin to get frustrated and discouraged. And even though you were happy with yourself just a moment ago, it all fades away when you see something better.

Social comparison is typical to an extent. According to some research, comparing yourself with others can be a vital source of motivation and direction. Our culture is littered with messages of what someone should strive to be, but unfortunately, these messages are not always reasonable or realistic. Instead of comparing apples with apples, we compare oranges with apples.

The man with the toned abs you are comparing yourself with most likely inherited a different body type than yours, so he builds muscle more easily or burns out fats faster. The images or success stories you see people share online and offline are often filtered to look perfect. Constantly making unrealistic comparisons between yourself and others might leave you with feelings of failure, damaging your self-worth. The comparison also causes you to focus more on others rather than yourself, making you feel you are not doing enough. Remember, this journey is for you and no one else. When you start worrying about not getting what the other guy has, you set off an inward feeling that can spiral down into anxiety and self-doubt. Moreover, comparison with others can negatively affect your relationships with friends and workout buddies. Being envious of one another's accomplishments makes it nearly impossible to support each other and genuinely celebrate when you reach milestones.

Entertain varieties in your workout

Doing the same thing, again and again, can be tedious and tiring. You need to spice up your game for some entertainment in your training. Our brains naturally crave varieties. If you have been doing the same old workout, you should consider stretching yourself. Think about some wild ideas that sound appealing and safe to you. You could perhaps take up a sport as a hobby. See if you can get a place to rent kayaks and look for local outdoor clubs you can go kayaking with some others. Anything you decide to do in this regard, make sure it's safe for you.

Even if your new workout isn't proving very challenging, give yourself some time to adjust to the recent activity your body is enduring.

Be self-disciplined

We all tend to be aware of the concept of discipline, but only a few of us truly understand what it entails. Successful people exert discipline daily. It is crucial to all of us, and without it, there would be chaos everywhere. Self-discipline is a form of freedom, freedom from lethargy and laziness, freedom of the demands and expectations of others, freedom from trying to satisfy others at the expense of your convenience, freedom from doubts and fears, release from instant gratification, and many other things. To train effectively and achieve maximum results, you need to show discipline. It requires lots of strength, not giving in to something you crave. It also takes lots of discipline to carve out time to train and be consistent with yourself.

Be patient

Mike Boyle once gave an analogy on training, "Training is like farming. You do all these things today that you can't see producing a result in the hope of a future payoff. You plant the seeds, water and fertilize, and scare away the birds, all in the hope that one day some little green shoots will pop through the soil."

You don't plant a seed today and expect to see results on the same day; the results are internal for some time. That's the same with strength training. It takes time. When these shoots start showing, that's when those who haven't seen you in a while tell you how great you look or ask you if you lost weight. Examining yourself in the mirror every day, you may not notice anything significant for a month or two, but with patience and consistency, the results start showing. You feel healthier; muscles become more visible, you get faster, stronger, and fitter. And life seems a little bit better.

Pay yourself

Anything with a valuable reward gets done by someone. Do you know why people do various jobs instead of us all doing the same thing, even the very strenuous ones? Take, for example, waste collectors. As I'm sure you all know, the job of a waste collector is to go around the assigned area and collect the waste for residential, commercial, industrial, or other. A rather thankless job that requires a strong stomach, if you know what I mean. So why would anyone offer their time to do such a difficult job? It's because they get paid - a fairly generous amount. In the U.K, waste collectors can earn up to £45,000 a year, depending on location. For reference, that's $62.500 in the U.S.; all they need is a school degree. With these salaries, there will never be a shortage of waste collectors, regardless of the job its self. Being rewarded for hard work is a powerful incentive and motivator. I want you to use this powerful motivator the next time you pass a milestone, even if it's a small one. Reward yourself by doing something you love, and I promise you personal drive will go through the roof.

A review of 11 randomized studies involving about 1,500 people found that using money as an incentive makes people more likely to exercise and be consistent for up to six months and even more. Also, how the financial incentives are structured influences the effectiveness. In a study, researchers gave 280 people the goal of reaching 7,000 steps every day. The subjects were randomly assigned to one of four groups: people in the first group got $1.40 every day they went 7,000 steps, which was $42 in a month; people in the second group were eligible to win a lottery prize of $1.40 every day they reached 7,000 steps; people in the third group got $42 in their account upfront, with $1.40 deducted every day they failed to reach 7,000 steps; the fourth group served as a control with no incentive. After 13 weeks, the winner was the group that had received money upfront. What's significant is that the threat of losing $1.40 every day was a more powerful incentive than the hope of earning it. Scientists who study economics and decision theory call this phenomenon "loss aversion": As much as we love receiving money, we hate losing it even more.

How can you apply this technique to motivate yourself? One way you can do this is to give an amount of money each month to someone; it can be anyone you trust to hold your money. For every month you are faithful with your workout sessions, you get your money back and expend it on a reward such as tourism or something you have wanted to buy. But if you fail to meet up, the person holding your money gives it away, maybe to your wife or kids, as pocket money. Or you could design one way yourself. However you decide to do it, it's an effective motivator when there's an incentive at stake.

Hopefully, now you have an idea of the mental fortitude it takes to embark on this journey. It's going to take some willpower at first, but if you can withstand the early storm, there is a sunny waiting for you ahead.

2

THE SECOND KEY

BUILDING YOUR FOUNDATIONS

I f you intend to build a house, the first thing you should do is sit down and analyze the cost, whether you have enough to finance your project from start to finish. If you fail to take this step seriously and go through the process without care and attention, you will find yourself in a situation where the house cannot be finished, and you have wasted all of your time. People might say, "This man began to build and was not able to complete."

Those words above were the words of Jesus Christ, written in the Bible. Whether you follow Jesus Christ or not, it doesn't matter. Achieving success starts at the very beginning of the journey. You are beginning your strength training program and want to be committed throughout the entire process because there is great satisfaction in having a plan and achieving it to the end. It propels you forward and motivates you to achieve even more.

Many beginners would love to have foresight into their program, see how well they will progress, or perhaps wish to have attained some progress already, but unfortunately, that is impossible. You don't start a journey in the middle. You start at the beginning and must endure what lies ahead of you.

One of the problems you may face before taking your first steps is the many challenging questions that will want to prevent you from ever starting in the first place. Questions like "Can I do this? How will this make me look to others? What if I have to spend lots of money? Can I see this through?" All these questions can paralyze you and even keep you from starting your strength training program.

That's why it's crucial to count the cost at the beginning. Measuring the price of taking on a new hobby helps you develop a blueprint for what is ahead. Blueprints help answer the difficult questions by giving you direction. They allow you to see the big picture and fill in the small details. Following a blueprint gives you the hope that you can get your desired result if you follow every step. The hope to think there is already a proven method for getting from point A to point B. If you follow the established plan, you'll have a greater likelihood of success than if you branch out on your own. And that's why I'm here to give you everything you need to start. Only make sure not to ignore this blueprint made for you through care and attention, just like a house.

What do you need to start your training?

Many people might recommend that you start by hiring a personal coach. But the truth is most people don't have the time or the money to invest in something like that. If you purchased this book, then I'm confident that you believe in the power of being self-taught and independent, not having to rely on someone else for your success. I admire you for this because it takes bravery to learn something the hard way. So let's just skip the personal trainer part and move on.

Most gyms have several resistance training machines and free weights such as barbells and dumbbells, but you can get a thorough strength training workout at home with or without equipment.

You don't need weights to build your lean muscle mass and tone your body. Don't disregard the multi-use tool given to you for free. I am referring to your own body. Your body weight is all you need to provide resistance for some strength training exercises like push-ups, squats, lunges, and many more.

However, if you desire to get some fancy new toys, you can do so with the following equipment but just remember, it's not necessary:

Dumbbells

We all know about these. They are the celebrities of gym equipment. Dumbbells are a brilliant place to start if you are new to strength training. Dumbbells are short bars with weights at each end. It can be used individually using a higher weight or in pairs simultaneously. Mostly all gyms are equipped with dumbbells ranging from 1kg to 50kg. They're friendly on your joints if used the right way and perfect for strength building. They allow your body to move naturally because your hands are not fixed to a position. I'll advise you to get adjustable dumbbells. This will allow you to add weights as you progress in your program. A beginner's set of 10kg adjustable weight dumbbells goes for an average of $50 - the price increases when you add more weight, understandably.

Barbells

Barbells are not just for athletes competing in a competition. Being the big brother to dumbbells, they can be lifters' friends for moves like deadlifts, back squats, and snatches. A barbell is like the longer, two-handed form of a dumbbell. It's a long metal bar to which weights are attached at each end. You can decide on the weight if it's an adjustable barbell, just like dumbbells. They allow you to add much more weight than dumbbells due to the strength of the bar. You can have as high as 20kg plates on each side of the metal bar. It would be best if you considered the weight of the metal bar too. Going between 15kg to 25kg is fair for you at the start. Do not purchase fixed barbells because you want to increase weight when training you progressively. Barbells are pretty expensive. An adjustable 50kg barbell could go for $200 on average so maybe save up a bit for that one. Remember, they are by no means necessary, and I will teach you workouts that don't require any equipment later on in this book.

Kettlebells

They are cannonball-like weights with a single loop handle. It's almost like the shape of a kettle, except it's got no spout. Like kettlebell swings and cleans, many classic kettlebell exercises require you to quickly and powerfully exert force on the weight. It's also a great way to work in some heart-pumping cardio. The weight of the kettlebell isn't balanced like a dumbbell; it shifts as you move it, this makes your body work harder to stabilize. It's excellent for training your balance. Considering you're over 50, kettlebells are great because they teach your body to adapt to the changing center of gravity. Just try not to fall over; I've made that mistake before. A 15kg kettlebell could go for $70 on average. Electric kettlebells, which are adjustable, are expensive and could go for over $250 on average.

Body Bars

The body bar is one of the simplest to use of all the strength training equipment, yet it is probably one of the least well-known. It's a slender long metal pole covered in foam rubber. It ranges in weight, making it a friendlier (and lighter weight) alternative to standard barbells. Body bars let you perform all kinds of exercises that you use barbells for, and they can be a good start for beginners. I recommend a 10kg body bar if you are a complete beginner. They are sold at around $50.

TRX

TRX stands for total body resistance exercise. It's a single piece of equipment made from two nylon straps suspended from the ceiling. You can use TRX to perform hundreds of strength training exercises, from push-ups to planks. TRX is an all-in-one tool. One of its most prominent benefits is dynamicity and versatility instead of an isolated movement. You will be working multiple muscle groups all at once. For instance, you can slip your feet into the TRX handles; your regular push-up turns into a core and shoulder-stabilizing move. And because you're using your body weight, you can adjust the resistance by moving your feet further (more resistance) or closer (less resistance) away from the anchor point. TRX could go for $40 on average.

Medicine Balls

They look a little like basketballs, but I don't think you could throw them that far. They are weighted balls, roughly the diameter of your shoulders. It's called a medicine ball because it also plays a vital role in sports medicine to improve strength and neuromuscular coordination. This ball-shaped weight can add resistance to core exercises like Russian twists or sit-ups.

You can also carry, lift or throw it. Moving medicine balls in several directions and planes of motion can involve more tissue, which helps lift energy use. A medicine ball could go for $25 on average.

Stability Balls

They are inflatable beach-ball-like strength training tools. They are helpful for bodyweight exercises that focus on the primary muscle that attaches the pelvis to the femurs (thigh bone) and spine. They can help you increase and improve spine stability through moves like back extensions and planks. This is very good for you if you spend a lot of time sitting at a desk. A 60cm stability ball could go for $15 on average.

Slam Balls

They are just like medicine balls. Although they are slightly larger and sometimes heavier, they don't bounce. It means you don't need to worry about the ball jumping into your face after you slam it. You can use slam balls to develop power, speed, and strength. Your muscles respond in proportion to how fast and powerful you slam the ball. A 10kg slam ball could go for $10 on average.

Resistance Bands

Resistance bands look like giant rubber bands. They are either flat or tubular. The different types of resistance bands may confuse you, but they fall under the same category. Although, they are used differently. They provide an effective workout. They are low impact and joint-friendly. Because the band creates resistance in both directions, your body is forced to remain stable. It will help you in training for balance. You can choose your desired resistance level, style, and length. You'll find everything from flat bands to tube bands with handles or even closed-looped bands. Try to get accustomed to their tension; at first, they might seem a little awkward, but you will get the hang of them over time. Resistance bands are perfect for exercises like squats, overhead press, and lateral band walks. This equipment is easy to move around, so you could even take them with you if you travel. Resistance bands are minimal in design and made out of cheap material, so you can typically get your hands on some for $15.

Sandbags

Just as the name describes, sandbags are weighted bags of sand; they look like big duffle bags. They are handy strength training tools made of durable materials. You can fill various materials inside them, not just sand. The materials you fill are known as fillers, and they're used for multiple functions while training. Although most people fill with sand, you can use pea gravel and rubber mulch. It's the best sandbag filler, in my opinion, because they don't make dust or pulverize. You can push your sandbag up, slam them down and slide them across the floor like a champ. Or, incorporate them into your strength training routine via squats, lunges, and carries. Sandbags will help improve functional fitness and get you ready for daily activities like carrying kids, bags of groceries, moving furniture, etc. And because the sand shifts as you move the bag, it helps challenge your wrist and forearm muscles, making them work harder to control the movement of the weight. Be sure not to fill your bag with more than 10kg for a start. Increase the fill as you progress in your training. You can get a moderate size sandbag for $10 on average.

ViPR

ViPR stands for vitality, performance, and reconditioning. ViPR is used to bridge the gap between movement and strength training. It combines full-body movement with load; hence, the name. ViPR builds mobility, stability, and dynamic strength through loaded movement training. Since you can pick it up and shift it in space, it mimics movements in sport and forces your body to work together. You can make forward lunges with rotation or lateral lunges while you swing the ViPR over and up as if you're using a shovel to dig. The ViPR can help you improve the strength and resilience of muscles and tissues, making it more resistant to many kinds of stain injuries. The muscles become lengthened under resistance and enhance the tissue's strength and density. The intensity of the movement can be altered based on how you hold the ViPR and how you move the tool to your center of mass. Pushing it further from your body makes it more challenging. ViPRs are pretty expensive... A 10kg ViPR could go for $200 on average. But don't worry, none of my teachings involve using these.

BOSU Balance Trainer

It is also referred to as a BOSU ball. BOSU stands for both sides utilized, which means you can use both the dome stability ball-like side and the flat side for exercises. It is like a stability ball cut in half. It consists of an inflated rubber hemisphere attached to a rigid platform. It is mainly used for balance training. You can use the dome side for exercises such as crunches on a softer surface that allows the full range of motion of the spine. You can stand on the flat surface to create a unique balance platform that helps engage lower body muscles. It's also perfect for building dynamic balance, enabling you to balance while in motion or change positions. A BOSU balance trainer could go for over $150 on average.

Gliding Discs

They are small, flat, two-sided round discs; one side is a fabric, and the other is hard plastic, or depending on your choice, both sides may have canvas-like material. You can use them on your feet and hands to provide a smooth gliding surface. Use these plate-size discs to crank up reverse or lateral lunges. You are sure to feel your core, glutes and inner thighs light up. They are also great for ab exercises like mountain climbers and pikes. Since you take resistance away from your feet, your core has to do all the work of stabilizing your body. A pair of gliding discs could go for only $10, so it's a good investment.

Parallettes

They are gymnastic tools, which are used in pairs. They are used to simulate the parallel bars found in professional gymnasiums. Much like push-up bars or dip bars, they are generally longer and lower to the ground. Gymnasts commonly use them. Parallettes allow you to test the limit of your physical strength. They allow you to perform exercises such as handstand push-ups, L-sits, and other gnarly feats of strength. And since you are raised off the ground, you can move into a deeper range of motion with each exercise. Parallettes could go for $60 on average, which isn't bad if you ask me.

Battle Ropes

If you want an intense and exhausting workout, try a workout with battle ropes. Battle ropes are used for fitness training to increase full-body strength and conditioning. They may not seem like much at first glance, but they provide a fantastic workout. Grab the rope with two hands and start lifting up and down to create waves or hold them in different hands for a more incredible exercise. The bigger the wave, the more energy you're putting into the rope. Try to keep the ropes moving fast. Using battling rope is like doing sprints for your upper body. They're perfect for fixing balance issues because you have to consistently put force into the lifts to keep that wave shape. Battle ropes could go for $40 on average.

The equipment listed above is all acceptable if you desire to have your strength training workout at home. You can enrich your home gym with several of the equipment listed. I suggest a dumbbell, body bar, resistance band, and perhaps, TRX. The prices attached above are just an average price to give you an idea of what it will cost you. Prices are mainly dependent on the brand of any of the equipment you're purchasing.

And don't forget you can register at a gym to get full access to a better range of equipment, including workout machines. Although, I do not advise fixed workout machines like smith machines because they restrict your body's natural movements.

TIPS FOR BEGINNERS

Warm-Up

You are over 50 and haven't trained before this time; chances are, your muscles are so alien to resistance training. Some aerobic exercises would do you so much good. It would help if you got involved in brisk walks or jogging for a day or two to prepare your muscles. This will increase blood flow to your muscles and prepare them for a good workout.

Start Moderately

If you're lifting weights, start with a weight that you can lift at least 5 to 8 times with proper form. Begin with 1 or 2 sets of 5 to 8 repetitions and progress with time. Nobody will make fun of you for using a smaller weight because everyone has to start somewhere.

Use proper form

Doing your workout in the correct form is vital. When lifting weights, use the full range of motion in your joints. Go through the movement in a slow and controlled manner, and this will also enhance the stress you put on your muscles. The better your form, the better your result, and the less likely you will sustain any injury. If you can't maintain good form, decrease the weight or the number of repetitions.

Rest In-between Workouts: Resting in-between workouts prevent muscle fatigues, especially as a beginner. Also, try not to hold your breath when lifting. Breathe out when you lift the weight and in when you lower it.

Limit your workout to a maximum of 20 minutes: Don't overdo it at the start. Remember, you might feel like your 30 still, but you have to consider your age. Twenty minutes will give you good results. With time you can increase it to 30 minutes.

Take note of pain

If your workout causes you pain, don't ignore it; stop immediately. Try doing the exercise in a few days or experiment with reduced weights.

Rest

Resting gives your muscles time to recover and replenish energy stores before the next workout.

Clothing

You can't work out without protecting yourself adequately. Get shoes and gloves suited for your workouts.

How to avoid injury during strength training

You must possess the correct form and body position when you engage in strength training. If you execute some of these exercises poorly, you can injure yourself. I have provided illustrations in the book to go with the exercises, but you can watch workout videos online to ensure you use the correct technique if you're unsure.

When you become comfortable lifting a particular weight, you can add about 5% of the current weight. But never rush things. The goal is to build, not to sustain injury. Be safe as best as you can.

3

THE THIRD KEY

ELITE BODYWEIGHT TRAINING

O ur muscle mass grows more and more depleted with each day.

As we grow older, physical fitness declines. More so as we grow over 50. Specifically, testosterone level decreases, weight typically increases, and the risk of contracting diseases or falling sick is grossly escalated. Regular physical activity like strength training plus proper nutrition and supplements are the central keys to combatting the inevitable effects of aging.

Prevention of injury, poor balance, and posture should be one of the main focuses of your strength training program. This chapter will discuss workout exercises you can do at home with no equipment, using just your body weight. Some people might be skeptical of a workout exercise that doesn't use any machine or external weight. But researches have proven bodyweight workouts improve strength and endurance. They are reliable exercises that anyone can do at any time. The problem I find people face is finding enough exercises to develop a complete routine. Not to worry, I have devised for you all of my top picks, covering all muscle groups.

BODYWEIGHT WORKOUTS

Bodyweight workouts are simple strength training workouts that use your body weight to provide resistance against gravity. They are effective ways to improve strength, balance, power, flexibility, endurance, speed, etc., all without the stress of buying equipment and learning how to use them. Bodyweight training uses simple abilities such as pulling, squatting, twisting, pushing, and balancing. Some of the standard bodyweight exercises include pull-ups, push-ups, and sit-ups, but there are many more.

If you are still not convinced, here are some of the benefits you will not find using weights or equipment.

Convenient: Using weights for a workout has benefits, but using your bodyweight surpasses dumbbells and barbells for convenience. You can achieve a blood-pumping and effective workout with your hands and feet anywhere you find yourself, whether that's at home or outside.

Efficient: You can change from one move to the next without expending time since no TRX, kettlebell, or ViPR is in the way.

With less rest, your heart rate maintains its elevated level, which is very important for burning calories. Bodyweight workouts are commonly done in interval training; you alternate between bursts of intense activity and periods of little or no intensity activity. This is proven to be more efficient than constant cardio.

Versatility: Squats and push-ups are perhaps the most effective exercises. Both are compound movements. They involve multiple joints and work on the most prominent muscle groups.

Customizable: Equipment limits you, but bodyweight exercises give you many options for any fitness level. It's just a case o discovering them. For example, the push-up can be done in various ways, from knees on the ground to clap and handstand push-ups.

No cost: Even though you can get your bodyweight workout done at a gym, all you will need is the floor beneath you, meaning you can do it at home, with no money spent on equipment.

THE TOP TIER OF BODYWEIGHT EXERCISES.

Hopefully, now you understand the usefulness of your own flesh. Let's dive into the exercises that I consider the best of the best. I will be describing these exercises, their benefits, and how to do them correctly, all of which have been carefully chosen for your age group, with injury prevention in mind. It can be hard to imagine the correct position of an exercise using only a bit of text on a page. To overcome this, I have provided illustrations of each activity that includes a starting position and a finishing position. They are numbered, so you can look back and refer to them at any time.

We'll start with workout exercises to work on the legs.

1. SQUAT

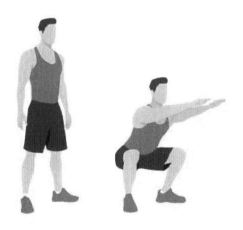

A squat is a strength exercise in which you lower your hip from a standing position while keeping your back upright. When you descend to squat, your hip and knee joints flex while your ankles dorsiflex (flexion of the ankle upwards). Conversely, your hip and knee joints extend, and your ankle joints plantarflex (extension of the ankle downwards) when you stand up. There are varieties of squats; we will be discussing the standard squat to keep things simple.

How to exercise:

- Pose: Before you squat, you should be in the proper squat position. Keep your feet a little bit wider than your shoulders. They shouldn't point straight ahead but will be turned out slightly depending on your comfort level between 5 and 30 degrees. This helps you keep balance.
- Maintain strong footing: Screwing your feet firmly into the ground help engage your muscles, improve alignment and create stability with the ground. It will also keep your arches from collapsing.
- Raise your chest: Your upper body matters as well. You have to keep your chest up and roll your shoulders back. Imagine an invisible pole passing from your lower back to the back of your head.
- Initiate the movement: When you're ready to squat, start the activity by bending your knees and pushing your hips back. Engage your core while lowering and keep it braced throughout the bend. Be sure to stay in control through the entire movement and go through it slowly. This will increase time under tension for your muscles, making them work harder. Inhale as you

bend down, and as you squat, your knees should be laterally above your toes, not reaching too inward or too outward.

- If you are looking for something to do with your arms, I suggest pointing them directly in front of you for extra stability.

- Stop when you reach a right-angle: You can bend lower to increase resistance, but it's acceptable if you stop when legs enter a right-angle position. If you have difficulty getting there due to lack of mobility or injury, then it's better to end the movement at any degree convenient and free of pain for you.

- Drive through your heels when you stand: Be sure to make your feet firmly on the ground throughout the time of your squat; You should focus on driving through your heels on your way back up. This will fire your posterior chain up, that's the muscles in the back of your body – your hamstrings and glutes. It would be best if you also exhaled on your way back up. Make sure to breathe throughout the move – breathe in on your way down and out on your way up.

2. LUNGE

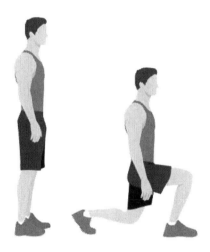

Have you seen a footballer knelt to tie a loosed lace while on the pitch of play? Or someone proposes on bended knee; then you are familiar with the lunge. A lunge is a single-leg bodyweight workout exercise that works your hips, quads, glutes, hamstrings and the muscles of your inner thighs. Lunges can improve endurance and lower body strength. When done the right way, they effectively target your lower body muscles without placing added strain on your joints. They are great moves for beginners.

How to exercise:

- Stand in a split stance with one of your legs forward and the other back. to get the proper length take one step forwards or one step backward.
- Ensure your torso is straight, and keep up on your toes for the back leg before you lunge
- Bend both knees simultaneously and lower your body until the knee at the back is about 3 or 4 inches from the floor.
- The front thigh should be parallel to the floor. Your weight should be shared equally between both legs.
- Push back up by straitening your front leg.
- Repeat for all reps before you switch legs.

Lunges can be very hard on your knees. The following tips are ways to make lunges easier on them:

- Be sure to keep the whole of your front leg foot on the ground.
- Remember the hips' role in performing a lunge. Keep your hip bones squared and facing forward, leading to more balanced training of the joints and muscles.
- Be sure to keep your rib cage over your pelvis; this will help engagement and better posture. Don't point your rib cage up. It could stress your low back. When your

rib cage is over your pelvis, you will breathe better and produce more power.

- Your front knee should align properly with your toes. Proper alignment is vital in lunges for joint health.

As an alternative or for variety, you can consider the side lunge. Start by standing upright with your feet shoulder-width apart. Take a big step to the side and make sure you keep your torso as upright as possible. Lower until you bend the knee of your leading leg at around 90 degrees while keeping your trailing leg straight, push back up to the starting position. An issue that may occur with the side lunge is collapsing over the straight knee. Focus on bending and lowering from the hips while your back is straight and core engaged, just as it is with a squat. Finally, be sure to keep both heels on the floor.

3. GLUTE BRIDGE

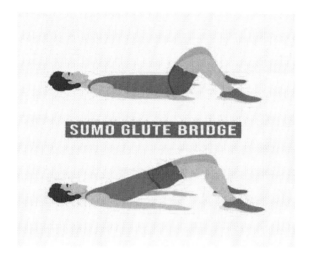

The glute bridge is a versatile, demanding, and effective bodyweight exercise. Regardless of your age or fitness level, the glute bridge is an excellent addition to any workout routine. It targets your hamstrings and glutes.

How to exercise:

- Lie on your back on the floor or an exercise mat. Bend your knees with both of your feet flat on the floor. Make your feet and knees in line with your shoulders. Contract your abdominal muscles to flatten your lower back into the floor. Make an effort to maintain a straight back throughout the exercise.
- Gently breathe out and engage your core while you pass your hips upwards off the floor into extension,

then squeeze your bottom at full extension. Make sure your feet are firmly pressed into the ground for more stability. Don't push your hips too high because this can generally increase the amount of arching in your low back.

- Breathe in as you slowly lower yourself back into your starting position.
- Gradually progress in this workout. After you've done several reps using both feet on the ground, you can move to the single-leg glute bridge. Remember not to push your hips too high to avoid arching that lower back.
- The single-leg glute bridge: lie on your back and bend your knees, so your feet rest flat on the floor, just as explained above. Then raise one of your legs and straighten it out. Then, repeat the normal movement of the glute bridge by driving your hips up while keeping the leg in the air straight.

4. FIRE HYDRANT

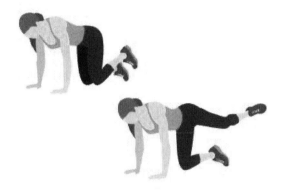

Also known as quadruped hip abductions. It's a bodyweight exercise that primarily works the gluteus maximus; some variations also work the core. The glutes control three major hip movements: hip extension, hip external rotation, and hip abduction. The fire hydrant involves all three actions. Performing this regularly will give you buns of steel. Having solid glutes improve your posture, reduce back and knee pains, and lower your risk of injury.

How to exercise:

- You start on all four – both hands and legs. With your hands under your shoulder and knees under your hips, as in a crawling posture. Make sure to keep your knees hip-width apart.
- Keep your hips level and core engaged, back flat, and

both legs bent at 90 degrees. Lift your leg out and raise it as high as your hip level; hold it for a second at this height.

- Lower the leg to return to its starting position. Repeat several times, then switch over to the other leg.

Do make sure to face the floor and avoid arching your back. Your elbows should be locked, and don't allow your weight to shift to one side. Take your time and try not to raise your leg above your hip. Breathe out as you raise your leg and in as you lower it.

5. STEP UP

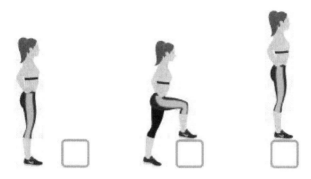

Just as the name suggests, it involves you stepping up to a higher platform and back down again. Step up is a simple body resistance exercise that works the leg and bottom muscles. It helps build strength in the quadricep muscles in the front of the thigh. Since the quads get little use in walking or running, it's a great way to balance this out. Building your quads also helps protect your knees. You can perform the step-up exercise anywhere as long as you have something stable to step on, for example, a bench.

How to exercise:

- Stand in front of a box or a chair, or you could use a step around you. Using your stairs at home is acceptable at first but keep in mind the higher the step, the more significant the resistance. So eventually, you will have to move on to something taller.
- Place any of your feet up on the step while the other is down. Press through your heel to straighten the leg.
- Bring the other foot to meet the one on top of the step.
- Bend the first knee on the step, and step down with the other foot.
- Bring the foot on the step down as well.
- You can repeat this for any number of reps, then change side and lead with the other foot while you repeat the sequence.

6. CALF RAISE

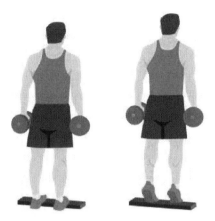

Most people tend to ignore their calves, but I am sure you don't want to be the guy looking like a popsicle stick when the shorts go on. It's not a good look. They are very instrumental to your daily life. Take, for instance, running or walking. For inactive people, calf muscles can be tight due to a lack of flexibility. To loosen up your calf muscles, try doing a bit of walking to warm up. The calf raise activates the muscles that run down the back of the lower leg: the gastrocnemius and soleus. These muscles are vital for ankle flexion and extension, propelling running and jumping. The gastrocnemius also works in alignment with hamstrings in the control of knee flexion. The soleus maintains proper balance and pumps blood from the legs to the heart.

When the calf muscles are weak, they easily cramp and strain, making walking and running difficult.

How to exercise:

- Spread your feet shoulder-width apart, then raise your heels slowly while keeping your knees extended. Pause for a second while you're stretched on your toes.
- Lower your heels slowly back to the ground.

Those are my top choices for the lower body based on science and research. Now let's move on to working your core.

7. CRUNCH

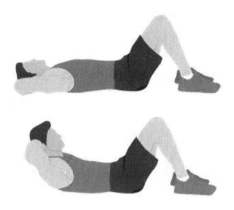

The crunch is a classic core exercise. It's a highly effective compound-muscle exercise for the abs. When you implement it correctly, it trains your upper and lower abdominal, oblique, and lower back muscles. These are the muscles that help stabilize your whole body. Crunches help you get a toned and ripped midsection and strengthen your stabilizer muscles like spinal erector muscles (your back). There are many benefits for the stomach, too; it helps people suffering from regular constipation by inducing bowel spasms and triggering its movement. A few minutes of moderate crunch session will also see you burning out lots of calories. But personally, my favorite part is the burn you feel when working the core. You will grow to love it!

How to exercise:

- Lie on your back on the ground. (You should use an exercise mat, which is more comfortable).
- Raise and bend your knees, and make your feet flat on the floor. Both knees and feet should be about a hip-width apart. Adjust your feet so that your heels are about a foot and a half from your tailbone.
- Cross both arms on your chest. You can also place your fingertips behind your head or neck if you're more comfortable with that.
- Lift your shoulder blades off the mat in a smooth and controlled motion. Breathe in, then breathe out as you engage your ab muscles and raise your torso. Lift yourself just enough to raise your shoulder blades off the floor. Once raised, pause in that position for a second or two. (You can have lower back strain if you lift your entire torso off the floor). Ensure your lower back, tailbone, and feet maintain contact with the floor.

- In a slow and steady motion, lower yourself back. Breathe in gently as you lower your torso gently. Smoothly controlling your movements work your ab muscles more effectively and help prevent injury. Always pause for a moment in between reps. If you rush the next rep, you will exhaust yourself lifting yourself instead of your muscles, leading to back injuries. The trick is to imagine just lifting your body with your abs. It helps if you keep them tensed throughout the motion.

8. FLUTTER KICK

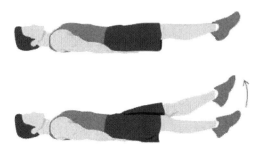

The flutter kick is an exercise that works muscles in your core. It specifically targets the lower rectus abdominal muscles and the hip flexors. Like swimming strokes, you can perform this move by lying on your back (or on your stomach if you want to strengthen your back muscles) and using your core to flutter your legs back and forth. Flutter kicks help improve posture, stability, and balance, improve endurance, and prevent injuries. It can also help burn calories and give more defined ab muscles.

How to exercise:

- Lie flat on your back and raise your legs to about 45 degrees. Keep your arms straight in line with the floor, or place them under your butt. You can lift your head, neck, and shoulders a little above the floor.
- While your legs are straight and glued together, start by lowering one leg.
- Raise the lowered leg and lower the other while focusing on keeping your core engaged.
- Continue the alternating movement between both legs.

9. RUSSIAN TWIST

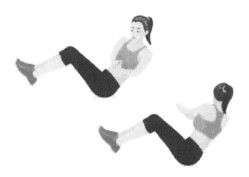

The final of our core exercises is the Russian twist. It's a valuable exercise that strengthens all parts of your abdominals, as well as your internal and external obliques, to give you a toned waistline and a more robust back. The twisting motion is the key to this move. It's a prevalent exercise among athletes as it helps with rotational movement, a valuable asset in sports. As you rotate with your abs from one side to the other, you fire up the muscle fibers around your waist and pull in the lower abs for a solid flat stomach. The Russian twist is a good calorie burner. It also helps improve balance and strengthen the lower back.

How to exercise:

- You start by sitting on your exercise mat, with your knees bent and feet flat on the ground.
- Then lean back so that your upper body is about 45 degrees off the floor. Make sure you keep your back straight at this angle throughout the exercise.
- Link your hands together in front of your chest, brace your core and raise your legs above the ground.
- Rotate your arms all the way over from one side to the other.

Now, let's move on to working out the back.

10. SUPERMAN

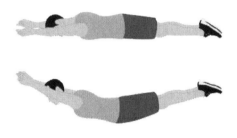

Undoubtedly, you must have seen Superman fly – either on a screen or in a picture. Today your gonna fly like Superman. However, you're flying will be achieved by lying on your exercise mat. The Superman strengthens your lower and upper back and your erector spinal muscles supporting the spine. Strong back muscles will prevent poor posture and discomfort. It also strengthens your glutes, hamstrings, and core. If you suffer from lower back pain or work at a desk most of the time, schedule the Superman in your workout. It's an excellent exercise to counterpart many core exercises.

How to exercise:

- Start by lying face down in a prone position, with your arms fully stretched backward and your legs stretched as well.
- Breathe out as you slowly lift your arms, legs, upper back, and head off the floor. Your body should have a slight curve, with your hands and toes some width from the ground.
- Hold your body in this pose. Then breathe out as you return to starting position.

11. REVERSE SNOW ANGEL

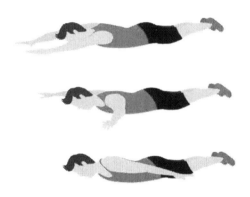

The reverse snow angel is a great exercise for improving strength. It also improves control of your scapular stabilizing muscles at its end ranges of motion.

How to exercise:

- Start by lying face down on your exercise mat, with your arms stretched out over your head and legs stretched out behind you.
- Lift your chest, arms, and legs a couple of inches off the floor. Move your arms backward to the pelvis and move your legs apart at the same time – just like trying to make snow angels.
- Return to starting position. That's a rep.

12. PLANK ROW

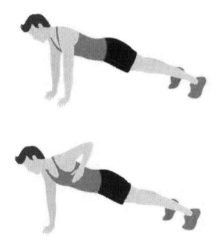

Plank Row is multifunctional. It requires your arms, legs, and ab muscles, making the exercise all-encompassing. Plank Row improves your posture by strengthening your back, chest, shoulders, neck, and abs, making it easier to keep your shoulders back and lower back in a neutral position. It helps your upper body rotation and improves balance. It challenges your core, increases stability throughout your spine, and trains the middle and upper back, shoulder, and arm muscles. Basically, anything you can think of, this exercise has got it.

How to exercise:

- Start in a plank position with your legs hip-width apart. Ensure your back is straight and your hands are stacked under your shoulders.
- Make your core tight and engage your glutes. Breathe out, stabilizing your torso as you lift one of your elbows to row, feel that side's shoulder blade sliding toward your spine as you bend your elbow toward the ceiling.
- Return the arm to the ground and repeat the movement for the other side.

The back has been ticked off the checklist. Next up... the chest.

13. PUSH UP

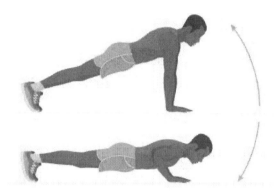

The push-up is one of the most common and popular workout exercises that are perfect for building the upper body and core strength. There is a reason why it's so popular, and it's because they are amazing. When you do it properly, it is a compound exercise that uses muscles in the chest, shoulders, triceps, back, abs, and legs to an extent. There are scores of variations of the push-up. As a beginner, you should start with leisurely versions and work up to the challenging ones as you progress.

How to exercise:

- Drop down to the floor and get into the press-up position. Your arms should be slightly lower than your shoulders and slightly out from them, with your fingers pointing forward.
- Stay balanced on your hands and toes. Let your body be in a straight line from your head to toes without arching your back or sagging in the middle. Your feet can be close or wider apart, whichever way is convenient for you.
- Contracts your abs and tighten your core before you start any moves. Make sure you keep your muscles are flexed throughout the entire push-up.
- Breathe in as you slowly bend your elbows and lower yourself until your elbows are at 90 degrees.
- Breathe out as you start contracting your chest muscles while pushing back through your hands to the start position.

As I've said, there are many variations of the push-up. I'll brief a few.

WIDE PUSH-UP

It is an effective exercise to build the upper body and core strength. It targets the chest and shoulder muscles more than the standard push-up, working the muscles on the ribs' surface beside the chest. All of this while providing support to the neck and back muscles. It is also beneficial for core stability, enhancing balance and posture, and protecting the back from injury.

How to exercise:

- Start in a plank position with your hands set wider than your shoulders. Your fingers should face forward.
- Bend your elbows out to the side as you lower your body toward the floor. Stop when your chest gets below your elbows.
- While in this position, engage your core as you press into your hands and lift your body back to the starting position.

DIAMOND PUSH-UP

It's also known as the triangle push-up. It's a compound exercise and a more advanced variation of the standard push-up. Diamond push-ups target and activate your triceps more than the traditional push-up. It's perfect for preparing your arms for other exercises such as pull-up or close grip bench press. It activates the chest muscles like the pectoralis major and shoulder muscles like the anterior deltoid as a compound exercise.

How to exercise:

- Start in a plank position. You can place your legs together or apart by a hip-width. The trick to this exercise is to connect your thumbs and index fingers to create a diamond shape.
- Engage your core and tuck your elbows against your body. Then bend your elbows as you push down your chest toward your hands until your upper arms are alongside your ribcage. Your shoulder blades should retract in the process.
- While you maintain proper form, return to the starting position by squeezing your chest and straightening your elbows. Your shoulder blades should protract as you return.
- On your way back up, squeeze your chest and triceps.

Incline Push-up: You should place your hands a bit wider than shoulder-width on a bench or box. With your feet rooted on the floor, bend your arms and go low until your chest touches the bench or box. Bring your body back up to the starting position and repeat.

Decline Push-up: You should place your feet on a bench or box with your hands rooted on the floor. Lower your body until your chest is almost touching the floor. Push your body back up to the starting position and repeat after a brief pause. It would help if you used a low box as a beginner.

There are many other variations of push-ups like the one-arm-push-up and clap push-ups. However, these are high in difficulty with few advantages to the previous variations. If I am honest, I think these techniques are often used to show off one's strength instead of building muscle. If you find the push-up too easy, you can always add more reps or add extra resistance using resistance bands. But don't worry, we will get into that later.

14. STAR PLANK

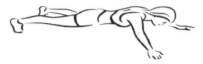

The star plank not only strengthens your obliques but your entire core. It builds strength in your shoulders and arms but deep contraction in your oblique muscles and hip. In addition, plank poses work on the strength of your mind and will because it requires a level of mental fortitude to maintain the position. It also offers you an opportunity to practice good breathing. Make sure you breathe well during this exercise.

How to exercise:

- From a push-up position, walk your hands and feet outward until they form an x-shape.
- Brace your core to keep a flat line from your head to your hips. And then from your hips to your feet.
- Stay in that position, then walk back to the standard push-up position.

15. REACH UNDER PLANK

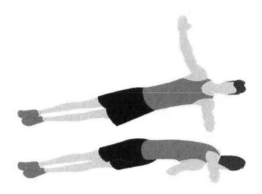

Plank reach primarily targets the abs and, to a lesser degree, the lower back, obliques, and shoulders.

How to exercise:

- Start in a plank position, put your hands under your shoulders, don't arch your back, and keep your core tight.
- Maintain the plank position. Lift one of your arms off the ground and touch the opposite hip with your hand. Return to the starting position and repeat for the other side.

Finally, we move on to the last but certainly not the least. Let's work on those arms.

The arms have always been considered the most difficult to get an effective workout only using body weight. Especially the biceps. This is far beyond the truth; people forget that we can create resistance in our limbs. The best part is you get to decide how much resistance you create! So, get ready as we prove all of the doubters wrong.

16. SIDE LYING BICEP CURL

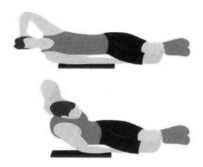

It might look weird, but the side-lying bicep curl is an excellent substitute for the bicep curl with weights. Although, it's not easy, and it requires some technique to practice the proper form for utilizing the movement effectively. It works the bicep muscles at the front of your upper arm and that of the lower arm: brachialis and brachioradialis. These are the muscles you use daily. Doing the side-lying bicep curl strengthens the upper arm and teaches you how to use your arm muscles.

How to exercise:

- Lie on any side; for this tutorial, we will say left. Then bend your knees and waist.
- Put your right hand behind your head.
- Grab your left leg with your left hand and pull on continuously while you flex your torso at the same time.
- Contract your bicep and hold for several seconds.
- Lower your body back down while keeping hold of your leg.

17. LEG BARBELL CURL

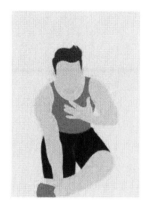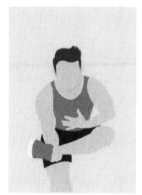

This bicep exercise is quite an easy one in base form. But remember, you can apply resistance by pushing against your arms with your legs. The more you drive away from your arms, the greater the resistance.

How to exercise:

- Begin this exercise by standing against the wall.
- Use your left hand to grab your right ankle with your palm facing upward.
- Lift your ankle towards your shoulder as high as you can, pause a few seconds, then lower it. That's a rep.
- Repeat for the other side.

18. COBRA PUSH-UP

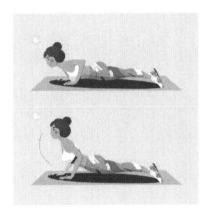

The Cobra push-up is a great bodyweight exercise for the triceps. It works on the hips, too, increasing the weight loaded through the triceps.

How to exercise:

- Lie on the floor with your chest and thighs flat on the ground.
- Place your palms on the ground, wider than a shoulder's width.
- Push the upper body up off the floor while keeping the lower half against the ground.
- Hold this position for 5 seconds and then lower back to the starting position.

19. BODYWEIGHT TRICEPS EXTENSION

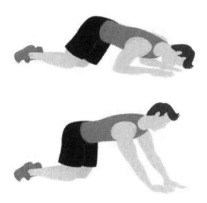

The bodyweight triceps extension is a calisthenics exercise that mainly targets the triceps and, to a lesser degree, the lower back and shoulders. There are many different variations you could do. Some require you use a barbell and squat rack. But that's not what this chapter is about, so we will be focusing only on your body weight.

How to exercise:

- You start on all four. Almost similar to the push-up starting position, only that your hands are a little forward and not directly under your shoulders. Stay balanced on your hands and toes.
- Slowly, bend your elbows so that you go low, and as against the regular push-up, you don't stop until your

elbows touch the floor and your hands form the L-shape.

- Return to starting position, and that is a rep.

That concludes my list of elite bodyweight exercises. Before moving on to the next chapter, I want to remind you that all of the listed activities have been chosen to provide you with the absolute best bodyweight training and to prove a point. That being, you can sustain a perfectly balanced training regime without spending a dime. That's the beauty of it. It is solely up to you how you exercise, and anyone can do it.

4

THE FOURTH KEY
THE ONLY EQUIPMENT YOU NEED

Strength training equipment is designed to assist and optimize fitness for users. They come in different styles and weights, as we've discussed some of them earlier. Fitness training equipment is costly, but they're a worthy venture in strength training and a daily reminder that you make a commitment to your fitness by spending money.

You've learned that you don't need weights to train, with over 20 workout exercises explained in the previous chapter. Now then, let's talk about how you can use equipment to build those muscles. We'll be discussing activities you can do with the dumbbell and resistance band only for this chapter. Unfortunately, we can't get everything in one book. But don't worry, I will be releasing another book for more experienced trainees, including you, once you have learned everything there is in this book! Dumbbells and resistance bands are more than enough to make staggering gains. Trying to use heavy weights or training with machines might be unsafe as a beginner. Even if you are familiar with strength training, it is better to master the basics and build a well of knowledge instead of going straight to the hard stuff with a puddle of information.

Dumbbells

You can achieve serious strength and mass goals by training with dumbbells. I'll even say, to fully maximize strength and hypertrophy, it helps if dumbbell training plays at least a partial role. This free weight is a handy and very useful workout tool. It's relatively small in size and inexpensive, suitable for a wide range of exercises you can perform from the comfort of your home. They're available in various types, shapes, weights, and materials, depending on your need. Owning a pair of adjustable dumbbells will undoubtedly help you save money from gym fees, yet you can still achieve your fitness goals. Let's look at some of the benefits of using this free weight for your workout.

Ease of training

It's effortless to train with a dumbbell. It doesn't matter who you are: old or weak; you can train with the dumbbell with ease. It also makes it easier for people with injuries to continue training without worsening the wound. If you have a shoulder injury, you won't be able to train your upper body using a barbell, but you can perform one-arm dumbbell training with the uninjured arm.

Increased Stability and Muscle Activation

A study compared the EMG activity of the chest, triceps, and biceps when performing a dumbbell bench press, barbell bench press, and Smith machine bench press. For reference, a smith machine is a gym equipment that assists you when exercising. It found that the dumbbell bench press and barbell bench press were similar in chest and triceps activity while the biceps activity was higher with the dumbbell - both higher than the smith machine. The reason is that using dumbbells requires so much stability, which activates more muscle fibers.

Removes Strength Imbalances: Dumbbells force the limbs to work individually. If one side is weaker than the other, the stronger side cannot cover the weakness of its pair, making dumbbells work on every imbalance in your arms.

Better safety

If you make a mistake and miss while having a heavy squat or bench press with a barbell, it means you could sustain a severe injury. Although there is still a risk with training dumbbells, it is significantly lower due to the size and shape.

Range of exercises

Dumbbells provide a vast range of movements. Almost every barbell exercise you can think of can be performed with the dumbbell. On the other hand, there are many exercise variations that the dumbbell will perform that won't be possible using different equipment, such as the single-arm and alternating arm exercises.

A final practical benefit of dumbbell training is that, in general, dumbbell exercises are less complicated to teach compared to other equipment exercises. For example, most strength training coaches, along with myself, agree that, on average, it is much easier to teach someone how to correctly use dumbbells than to teach that same person how to use a chest fly machine. This means you can swiftly get through the teaching process and move on to the fun stuff like getting those reps in and watching your muscles blow up.

RESISTANCE BANDS

Resistance bands are giant rubber bands. Mixed in with your bodyweight exercises, they produce the ultimate combo, a partnership that can shoot you straight to the top of your goals. There are different kinds of resistance bands. The most common ones are the three flat resistance bands, also known as strength bands or exercise bands. You can get them in different sizes. The thicker the width, the more resistance it gives and the harder it is to stretch. Resistance bands typically start at level 1 and go all the way up to level 6: the same length but with a different level of resistance. A level 1, as I'm sure you have guessed, is easier to stretch. It's better suited to exercises that involve a great range of motion or some other resistance like a bodyweight exercise. And since it's slightly easier to use, it is the ideal choice if you are just starting out. Unlike dumbbells, they are practically weightless, so they become very portable; fold them up and put them in your bag. That's all it takes to have a killer workout wherever you are. They're also very cheap, one of the most affordable among strength training equipment. Now, let's talk about some benefits you get when you train with the resistance band.

Improves the quality of your exercise: When you train with a resistance band, the activity is entirely different than if you were using a weight. Instead of simply lifting a weight, the band puts your muscles under constant tension. There's more contraction as your muscles work harder. This makes the actual quality of each rep to be significantly improved.

Recruits your stabilizing muscles: Resistance bands will make you feel a bit unsteady because they tend to wobble, forcing you to work more to maintain form. As you do this, you're targeting the stabilizing muscles and building core strength all at once.

Works compound exercises: Compound exercises are exercises that use and work several muscles simultaneously. Resistance band exercises are naturally more inclined toward compound moves so that you can use them for a full-body workout.

Promotes better form: Often, you would have to exert a lot of momentum to squeeze out the last few reps while doing a particular exercise. It is much harder to do when you use resistance bands. Having to cope with the instability of the bands will force you to perform the movement correctly so that you don't disrupt the distribution of weight.

Offers safety: Your safety is paramount. As I've once said, your goal is to train, not sustain injury. Even when you are alone, resistance bands offer strength training with no risk of dropping a heavy weight on your body or crushing your fingers between weight plates. That makes them more suitable for working out when your alone or don't have someone else training along with you.

Now you can see that the dumbbells and resistance bands are great tools with lots of benefits, even if they look simple. So, let's dive into some exercises you can do with this equipment and learn how to use them. For all the dumbbell exercises, start with a lightweight dumbbell. You will add to the weight as you progress and gain more stability and strength. It's all about listening to your body. Unfortunately, I can't tell you when to increase more weight because I don't know you. The one who knows you best is yourself, so listen to your body, and if you think it's time, then it most likely is.

1. DUMBBELL GOBLET SQUAT

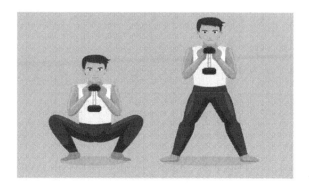

This is one of the safest and most effective weighted squat exercises. It will help you build impressive leg and glute strength. It primarily works the quadriceps and the glutes. When the quadriceps muscle is activated, hypertrophy in these muscle cells is increased dramatically. Plus, the glutes receive a good amount of tension during the dumbbell goblet squat. This exercise also secondarily works the core, hamstrings, calves, and arms. As you perform squats, your core does the duty of stabilizing your body to maintain balance; your hamstrings and calves also get worked to reinforce your legs and your arms contract as you stabilize the dumbbell.

How to exercise:

- Start by holding a dumbbell vertically with both hands holding onto the top end of the weight.
- Stand with your feet about shoulder-width apart. Try to engage your core and keep your back straight.
- Bend your knees and lower your hips towards the floor.
- When your hips are straight in line with your knees, pause, then contract your quads and glutes.
- Return slowly to the starting position.

2. LUNGE WITH DUMBBELLS

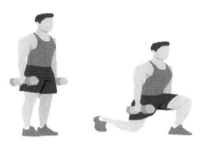

A lunge with weights such as dumbbells gives additional work for the upper leg muscles and the glutes. Lunges with weights require good balance. If you have balance issues, start the exercise without weights while learning the proper form in the process. Regular lunges are number #2 in the ELITE BODYWEIGHT TRAINING chapter if you need to refer back to it. This exercise mainly targets the quadriceps muscles at the front of the thigh. To a lesser degree, the gluteus maximus of the butt, adductor Magnus of the thigh, and the soleus of the calf. Muscular quads help you maintain balance and mobility.

How to exercise:

- Stand upright with one dumbbell in each hand. Place your arms at your sides. Your palms should be facing your thighs. And feet should be shoulder-width apart.
- Take a big step forward with any of your legs. Bend the other knee until the front thigh is parallel to the ground. Breathe in as you go down.
- Step back to your starting position while you breathe out.
- You should have all reps for a side before changing to repeat for the other side.

3. DUMBBELL BENCH PRESS

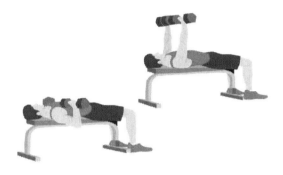

As a beginner, you shouldn't even attempt bench presses with barbells. Instead, it would help if you considered using the dumbbell as a fantastic variation of the bench press workout. Using dumbbells allow for a complete range of motions, which lets you work the pec muscles to their maximum. This exercise does absolute wonders for your pectoral muscles, and as a bonus, it works your triceps too. Using a dumbbell will also mean you train different sides independently; a weak side won't depend on the other to suffice for its weakness. This means no muscles get left behind!

How to exercise:

- Lie on your back on a bench holding two dumbbells, one in each hand, just to the side of your shoulders. Your palms should face your feet in the starting position.
- Lift the weight above your chest by extending your elbows until your arms are straight. However, try not to lock your arms when they are straight because this will take pressure off the muscles and onto the joints, which you don't want.
- Bring down the weights slowly back to the starting position.

4. BENT OVER DUMBBELL ROW

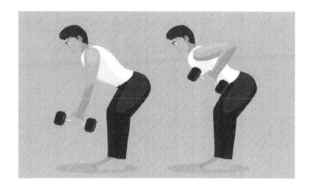

It's a variation of the bent-over row, an exercise to build your back muscles and strength. Your back muscle requires some amount of variation. So, it's acceptable to experiment with several angles and hands positions to maximize your back muscle growth. Rows are essential to training for balanced muscle growth and strength. Use the dumbbell bent-over row when you are training your back, and it will be a great attention to your workout.

How to exercise:

- Stand while you hold a dumbbell in each hand with a neutral grip. Before bending over, it is vital to stabilize your back. To achieve this, make a slight bend in your knees and stick your bottom out as you bend with a straight back - kind of like how a gorilla stands.
- Hinge forward until your torso is almost parallel with the floor, and start the movement by driving your elbows behind your body while you retract your shoulder blades.
- Pull the dumbbells towards your body until your elbows are at midline with your body.
- Slowly lower the dumbbells back to the starting position under control.

5. DUMBBELL BICEP CURL

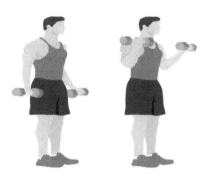

In my opinion, the most common and most fun exercise on this list. The bicep curl primarily works the upper arm muscles, and to an extent, the lower arm. You make use of these muscles all the time in day-to-day business. It's a great exercise for strength and muscle definition. This exercise gives you sculpted arms and makes you better at other exercises like rows where your biceps work to pull weights back to your body. Dumbbell bicep curls also involve a lot of stabilization; it will help train your shoulders to be more stable and teaches your core to engage.

How to exercise:

- Start by standing in a neutral position with your feet shoulder-width apart. Make sure your abdominal muscles are engaged.
- Hold one dumbbell in each hand, relax your arms down at the sides of your body with your palms facing inward.
- Let your upper arms remain stable and your shoulders relaxed. Bend at your elbows, lift the weights; make sure that the dumbbells approach your shoulders. Try to keep your elbows tight to your rib cage and make your biceps do all the work, not your entire body. Breathe out while you lift.
- Lower the weights back to the starting position. Breathe in while you lower the weight. Try not to drop the weight down. It's a bad habit people get into. Lifting the dumbbells is only half the exercise; the other half is bringing them down again using the muscles in your biceps.

6. CROSS-BODY DUMBBELL HAMMER CURL

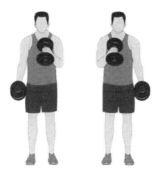

You lift the weight across your torso rather than lifting in front of your body. This exercise does not work only your biceps but also your brachialis and brachioradialis. It increases muscle mass in your biceps and significantly in your forearms. It also creates a balance between the upper and lower regions of the arms. In other words, this was Popeye's favorite exercise.

How to exercise:

- Hold a pair of dumbbells, one in each hand, by your sides.
- Stand upright with your palms facing towards your body.
- Slowly start to curl one dumbbell up across your body to the opposite shoulder. Make sure your palm is facing inward, and squeeze the bicep at the top position.
- Pause for a second and slowly lower back to the starting position. Repeat for the other side.

7. DUMBBELL SIDE LATERAL RAISE

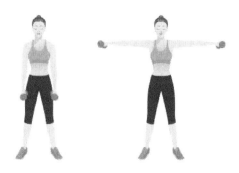

The side lateral raise is an effective exercise designed to strengthen the shoulders. With a pair of dumbbells and enough shoulder flexibility, you can build stronger and broader shoulders with ease. This exercise primarily targets the lateral head of the deltoid, enabling isolation of these muscle groups. Although, it also engages the posterior and anterior heads but not as drastically. If you do this exercise regularly, you can achieve hypertrophy (an increase of muscle cells) of the lateral deltoid, which gives the appearance of broader and firmer shoulders. Aside from the appearance benefits, the shoulder joints are the most unstable in the body; sufficient strength training designed to target them can help keep your shoulders healthy and fit. The shoulders are also one of the most neglected primary muscle groups, so if you're looking for that edge, this exercise with give you a huge advantage.

How to exercise:

- Stand upright, with one dumbbell in each hand. Your arms beside you with your palms facing inward.
- Place your feet about hip-width apart.
- Raise your arms laterally at the same time, try to keep them straight as you raise them, stop when your elbows reach shoulder height so that your posture forms a 'T.' Breathe in as you lift.
- Pause and hold at the top for a second before lowering back to starting position slowly. Breathe out when you lower the weights.

8. DUMBBELL SHOULDER PRESS

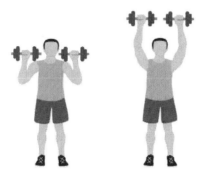

The dumbbell shoulder press is one of the few exercises that can produce muscle mass, strength, and giant boulders as shoulders. Its movement is similar to the strict press (barbell) with significant growth of the shoulder, triceps, and upper chest. This exercise increases strength throughout the shoulders and engages the core for stability. You can perform it both standing and sitting, with your dumbbells held horizontally at your shoulders or rotated in a hammer grip. When you complete it sitting down, it stabilizes your back.

Conversely, it works a more expansive range of muscles from the standing position. It works in all aspects of the deltoid muscles of the shoulder. This one is up to you whether you perform it standing up or sitting down, but keep your personal goals in mind when deciding.

How to exercise:

- Stand (or sit) upright and keep your back straight.
- Hold a dumbbell in each of your hands with your elbows at shoulder height, forming a 90-degree angle while maintaining a sturdy grip. Your thumbs should be inside, and your knuckles should face up. That's your starting position.
- Raise the dumbbells above your head in a controlled motion while you breathe out.
- Pause at the top of the moment. Return the dumbbells to your shoulders while you breathe in. That's a rep.
- Keep the dumbbells slightly in front of your shoulders, so there isn't pressure on the rotator cuffs.

Use extremely light-weighted dumbbells if you are a beginner to avoid injury because, as explained earlier, your shoulder joints are a little weaker, so you need to take caution. You will add more weight as you progress.

9. OVERHEAD DUMBBELL TRICEPS EXTENSION

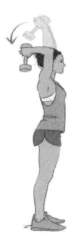

You can also work the triceps extension exercise while standing, sitting, or even lying down. Overhead dumbbell triceps extension requires you to move your triceps through a full range of motion to work them properly. It's a move that isolates the triceps and not much else. The benefit of this is that your triceps have to work extra hard because they aren't getting any help from the other muscles, meaning they have elevated levels of growth. If your body is looking great, but you know your triceps are severely lacking, this is the one for you.

How to exercise:

- Start by standing with your feet placed apart by a shoulder width. Hold a dumbbell with both hands in front of you.
- Raise the dumbbell over your head until your arms are almost straight. That's your starting position.
- Slowly bend your arms to lower the dumbbell back behind your head. Be mindful of your elbows; try to keep them inward. If they go too far out, it incorporates your biceps too much. Once your forearms go past a 45-degree angle, bring the dumbbell back to the starting position. That's a rep.

Like in the overhead dumbbell press, use highly light-weighted dumbbells at the beginning if you are new because this exercise puts a tremendous amount of stress on your triceps.

10. ONE-ARM DUMBBELL ROW

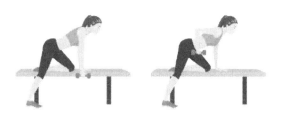

If you want to build a solid back, then the one-arm dumbbell row should be in your wheelhouse, especially for the fact that there's no shortage of variations for you to choose from. Although the bent-over barbell row is the most common, and it's worth its hype due to the massive back-boosting benefits it provides. Yet, it's fair to say that the one-arm dumbbell row is better for your back than the bent-over barbell row. This is because using just an arm lets you focus your efforts on the lats, traps, and the other back muscles this exercise targets. Also, using dumbbells instead of a barbell prevent strength imbalance because (as previously stated) your strong side could be covering up for the weakness of the other. Furthermore, A single-arm with a dumbbell has a greater range of motion than the bent-over row.

How to exercise:

- Get a bench or a sturdy thigh-high platform that you can lean on when doing the exercise. Place your left knee on the platform and place your left hand palm-down on the bench to gain balance. It would help if you had your dumbbell already set on the floor to one side so that you don't have to get out of position to retrieve it.
- Your back should be parallel to the ground while on the bench. Reach down with your right hand for your dumbbell, pick it up with a neutral grip, your palm should be facing you.
- Slowly pull the dumbbell up to your chest, concentrate on lifting it with your back and shoulder muscles rather than your arm. Let your chest be still as you lift. Squeeze your shoulder and back muscles at the top of the movement. Then lower the dumbbell until your hand is fully extended.

11. DUMBBELL RUSSIAN TWIST

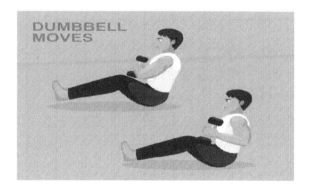

The Russian twist is an effective exercise that strengthens all parts of your abdominals, as well as your obliques, to give you a toned waistline and a more muscular back. The twisting motion is the key to this move. We discussed the regular Russian twist in the previous chapter but adding a dumbbell puts more pressure on you as you twist. As you rotate with your abs from one side to the other, you fire up the muscle fibers around your waist and pull in the lower abs for a solid stomach.

How to exercise:

- You start by sitting on a mat (or the floor if you don't have one), with your knees bent to an angle where your feet can comfortably lay flat on the ground, holding a dumbbell with both hands in front of your chest.
- Then lean back so that your upper body is about 45 degrees to the floor. Make sure your back straight at this angle throughout the exercise.
- Brace your core and raise your legs above the ground.
- Slowly twist all the way over from one side to the other with the dumbbell.

Believe it or not, we've exercised every part of the body using the dumbbell – the leg, back, core, biceps, triceps, chest, and shoulder. Now that your knowledge is vast in dumbbell training, we can move on to the final set of exercises for this book. If you haven't already, I suggest you buy yourself some resistance bands because the rest of this chapter will be devoted to them.

12. RESISTANCE BAND SQUAT

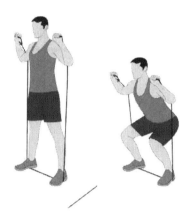

Resistance band squat is a lower body exercise that uses the band's resistance to give more strength to your legs and glutes. It's a move that offers added benefits to your regular squat. First, you must know how to do the standard squat (explained in detail in chapter 4 exercise #1). Then, grab a band, and now instead of doing 20 squats, you only have to do 10 to get the same result. This exercise is a unique way to strengthen and tone your glute muscles. Many people don't have their glutes worked adequately in the typical squat exercise. Using the band gives you the power needed, allowing you to sit back on your heels to concentrate on working your glutes for the motion. In addition to the excellent work on your glutes, your quads and hamstrings get strengthened as well. Your muscles get involved as you press up to standing against the force of the band.

How to exercise:

- Stand on the band with your feet placed shoulder-width apart. Hold the handles next to your shoulders, which puts the band behind the back of your arms.
- Slowly, sit down back into the squat position while keeping your abdominals tight and chest lifted.
- Press back up through the heels, squeezing your glutes.

13. RESISTANCE BAND BICEP CURL

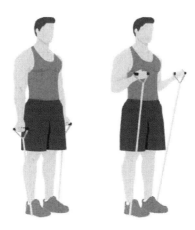

This exercise strengthens your biceps without the use of any weight. It uses the band's resistance to engage your biceps and contract them. If you have injuries in your wrists that prevent you from holding equipment like the dumbbells, consider the resistance band bicep curl. The resistance band challenges you to work against the pulling force of the band rather than using weights against gravity. Like most bicep curl exercises, it works your biceps to strengthen the muscles, and with the variety of resistance levels, you can personalize this technique.

How to exercise:

- Stand on the band with both feet, holding the handles long next to your sides with your palms facing forward.
- Slowly, curl your hands towards your shoulders. Squeeze your biceps as you do this and keep your elbows next to your side, just like a dumbbell curl.
- Slowly un-curl your arms back down to starting position.

14. RESISTANCE BAND OVERHEAD TRICEPS EXTENSION

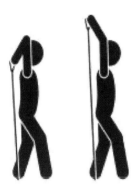

This is an upper-body exercise that focuses mainly on your triceps. It helps isolate the triceps muscle and avoid cheating with different body parts. Overhead triceps extension with a resistance band is a super effective exercise for working the back of your arms. It's a similar exercise to a gym using a cable machine. The angle of your body in this exercise is optimal since your body weight can offset a more incredible amount of resistance. The hidden bonus to using a resistance band for your overhead tricep extensions is that it's the only one that makes your arms work independently, unlike the dumbbell and cable machines that pair your arms together. Couple this with the fact you're doing an exercise that isolates the triceps means that you better get ready for that burn because it's coming.

How to exercise:

- Stand with one foot slightly in front and place the center of the band under the foot at the back. Or you could take a step back; it doesn't matter as long as the band wraps around the back foot.
- Bring the handles straight up above your head. Your elbows should be pointing in front of you.
- Slowly, lower handles behind your head until your elbows bend at 90 degrees, keep your elbows close to the side of your head.
- Slowly, press your hands back up overhead.

15. RESISTANCE BAND PULL-APART

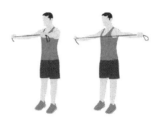

The resistance band pull-apart is a simple exercise but a great one. Its movements strengthen the muscles in your upper back and the stabilizer muscles in your shoulder joints. Building these areas improves your posture and increases your bench press, squat, and deadlift capabilities.

How to exercise:

- Stand with your arms stretched out directly in front of you, parallel to the ground.
- Hold your resistance band and grip it tightly with both hands.
- Keeping your arms straight, stretch the band apart by pulling both hands out to your sides. Use your mid-back to initiate this movement.
- Keeping your spine straight, squeeze your shoulder blades together like you're trying to squish a grape between them.
- Slowly return to the starting position.

16. RESISTANCE BAND BENT OVER ROW

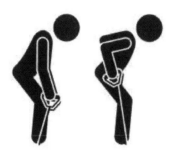

The bent-over row with a resistance band is an easy exercise to perform that primarily targets the middle and lowers back, and to a lesser degree, also targets the shoulders and biceps.

How to exercise:

- Start by stepping on a resistance band with your feet at shoulder-width apart, toes pointing out slightly.
- Bend your knees slightly and push your hips backward. Brace your core and back throughout.
- Leading with your elbows, pull the band's handles back, bringing your shoulder blade closer together. Hold this contraction and slowly release it back to the starting position.

17. RESISTANCE BAND SEATED ROW

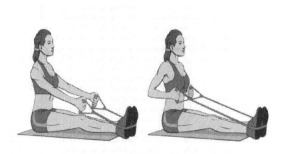

The seated row with a resistance band strengthens the upper back muscles. The upper back muscles give you balance when you train your chest muscles with exercises such as push-ups and chest presses. The upper back muscles enhance good posture and balance your body's muscles. Plus, the movement is nearly identical to using a rowing machine without coughing up 500 dollars.

How to exercise:

- Hook the middle of the band to a stationed object at ankle height.
- Sit on your exercise mat and grasp the handles, your palms facing each other, and your knees slightly bent. If you don't have handles, just wrap the bands around your hands. Keep your posture erect and lower your back slightly arched.
- Slowly, pull the handles to your lower back abdomen while your elbows are close to your sides.
- As the handles touch you, squeeze your shoulder blades together and then reverse direction, returning slowly to the start position.

18. RESISTANCE BAND PUSH-UP

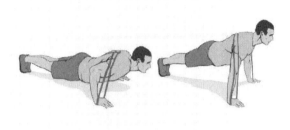

If you intend to increase the challenge of your push-up, then the resistance band is a way to go. They ideally intensify push-ups because you rely on all the muscles in your upper body to lift your body weight against the band's resistance. Doing the resistance band push-up will work the muscles in your arms, chest, back, and core.

How to exercise:

- Wrap the band around your back right under your armpits while holding the handles. Loop the band around each hand again to tighten it.
- Kneel down while you place handles against the floor, then extend your legs long until you are in a plank position.
- Slowly lower your chest to the floor while keeping your body long. Press back up until arms are fully extended.

19. RUSSIAN TWIST WITH RESISTANCE BAND

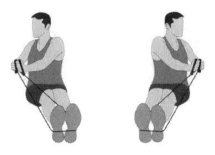

Russian twist specializes in developing your obliques and your general core strength too. Doing the exercise with a resistance band is an excellent option because you keep your legs suspended, which creates more force acting on your obliques; this trains them more effectively than doing it with just your bodyweight.

How to exercise:

- Wrap the band around your feet, grab one side of the band with each hand, and pull it up so that your hands are in line with your hips.
- Lift your legs off the ground.
- Make sure you chose a band with enough resistance, enough to feel its impact.
- Then lean back so that your upper body is about 45 degrees to the floor. Ensure you keep your back straight at this angle throughout the exercise.
- Brace your core and raise your legs above the ground.
- Slowly twist all the way over from one side to the other.

20. RESISTANCE BAND OVERHEAD PRESS

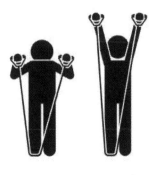

The resistance band overhead press strengthens the shoulder muscle and increases the stability in the body. Pushing the resistance of the band upward is done with the deltoid muscle. When you extend your body, you need to tighten your core and glutes, which increased stability throughout your body. When performing this exercise, keep your abdominals pulled in tight and slightly bend your knees.

How to exercise:

- Stand in the center of the band with both feet set apart by a hip's width.
- Bring handles of the band above your shoulders so that your elbows are bent 90 degrees.
- Press arms straight up, and just like the dumbbell shoulder press, remember to put your arms slightly ahead of your shoulders throughout the movement. Slowly lower your arms back to a 90-degree angle, then repeat.

21. WOODCHOPPER WITH RESISTANCE BAND

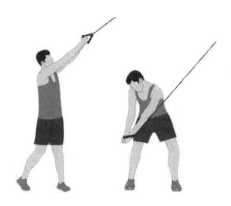

Woodchoppers are good exercises for tightening and toning the obliques. The abdominal muscles get most of the attention of the woodchopper. The woodchopper with a resistance band uses the band to simulate a wood chopping action. It's a compound pulling motion and a functional exercise. It builds strength and power in your core and obliques, imitating many sports activities like swinging a bat or throwing while you twist your torso. While it primarily targets the abdominals and obliques, the shoulders, back, and glutes also have a part to play in this exercise. This activity can be done from two different angles. The first is a movement going from your feet with resistance as you go upwards. The second is from a high place like between a door, pulling when you go downwards. I will teach you the latter because I believe it has the most benefits. However, it is my job to inform you of all options.

How to exercise:

- Anchor one end of the resistance band towards the top of a door and close it to trap the band in place. Test it before use to make sure it is tightly secured.
- Stand with your left side towards the door. Position your body so that the band movement will be downward and across your body as if you were planning on chopping a tree. Make sure your feet are in a comfortable position. Hold onto the free end of the band with your arms held towards the band.
- In one smooth motion, keeping your abs engaged, swing the resistance band across your body until it passes the opposite thigh. Don't be stiff; you should rotate your waist, hips, and knees slightly, all as one.
- At the end position, slowly allow the band to return to the starting position.

22. REVERSE CRUNCH WITH RESISTANCE BAND

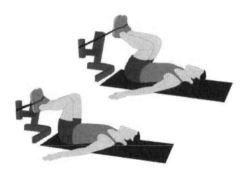

The key to a good and effective reverse crunch is moving in a controlled motion; we don't want to injure your back by making sharp movements. Your abs are kept under tension throughout the entire exercise. Adding a resistance band to the activity increases the pressure involved and gives the abs a lot more to deal with. The reverse crunch with a resistance band strengthens your rectus abdominis, which is the muscle that flexes your trunk and spine. It also targets and activates your transverse abdominis, the deep muscle below your abdominals, and your external obliques.

How to exercise:

- Anchor the band at the base of a pole and anything secure to hook on.
- Lie on your exercise mat, face up. Raise and bend your knees at 90 degrees.
- You can stick your hands to the mat to add stability wherever is most comfortable.
- Put both feet into both handles of the band, and scoot back to create tension.
- Make your abs tight and your back flat to the ground. Then, pull your knees towards your shoulders while you contract your abdominal muscles.
- Slowly return to the starting position.

23. RESISTANCE BAND CHEST PRESS

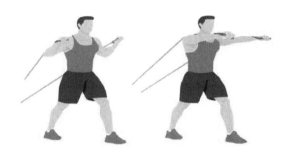

congratulations, you've reached the very last exercise in this book! Lastly, we will discuss an effective exercise for your arms and chest that doesn't involve getting down on the floor and doing a press-up. It uses the band's resistance to work in an opposing motion to strengthen your biceps, triceps, chest, and the front of the shoulder. It also teaches your body to engage the core for stabilization. The exercise is similar to the dumbbell or barbell chest press, but you can accomplish it from a standing position due to the band resistance. You might need to pick up a band with a high resistance level because the distance the band travels is relatively short.

How to exercise:

- Similar to the woodchopper, trap the resistance band in the door with two ends sticking out. Ensure it is properly secured.
- Take one step forward and bring the handles to your shoulders with your palms facing forward. Hold your elbows slightly behind your body.
- Stand tall with your abs tight, and concentrate on good posture through your spine. Roll your shoulders back to maintain good posture.
- Push your arms straight out in front of your chest and shoulders.
- Then, slowly pull elbows back to the starting position.

That concludes our list of exercises. Of course, there are many, many more, but after hours of research and years of knowledge in fitness, I truly believe these are the best for bodyweight, dumbbell, and resistance band training.

I hope the instructions I devised were clear enough, and you can start the next chapter full of confidence. If I could relay to you one last piece of advice, it would be to make sure you are squeezing the muscles you're trying to build throughout the entire movement. It may not seem like it's doing much, but it makes all the difference in the world. That is why I always suggest performing your exercises slowly and in a controlled manner so you can focus on putting pressure on your muscles.

5

THE FIFTH KEY

A PLAN FOR SUCCESS

Last month, my neighbor registered at her local gym, she went a couple of times a week for about three weeks, but that was the end. A relatively short-lived venture. I know this because I ran into her several weeks back near my house. We had a little friendly chat. We are reasonably close, and I remember telling me how excited she was to get back into fitness like she used to be during her early 20's. A few weeks later, I stopped seeing her leave the house with her gym clothes; since then, there hasn't been any mention of her regaining her fitness. Although it's not new to me, I've seen it countless times. People come to the gym, hop on the fun-looking equipment, have a wander about, and then you never see them again. The funny thing is, you can spot that type of person a mile away, just from looking at their tendencies, whether it's taking multiple gym selfies on their phone or putting minimal effort into each rep. Their lack of drive radiates off them like a nuclear powerplant.

Yes, it's okay that they made it to the gym in the first place. It's highly commendable. At least, a journey of a thousand miles begins with the first step. But failing to plan for the months ahead and a clear goal for the future often results in a lack of conviction.

There is a famous saying often credited to Benjamin Franklin, "failing to plan is planning to fail." This quote may just sound like a clever play on words to some ears because of its lyrical rhymes, but it's highly factual. Planning is a critical factor in every facet. When neglected, failure may be inevitable.

Having all the information about workout exercises, their benefits, equipment, and how to exercise is never enough if there is no solid plan to use this information for effective productivity.

A workout plan is vital if you are going to succeed in your fitness goals. It would bring me great joy if you saw it as the number one tool in the list of equipment you need for your strength training program. It is the tool that will help you to navigate through your work schedule and other obligations, keeping you motivated towards achieving your goals and assist in breaking down your step-by-step plan on how to attain them. I've gone into greater detail about the potential benefits you enjoy from having a workout plan.

- **It helps create a lifestyle:** A workout plan is a perfect way to form a lifestyle, more so, for older men. A plan makes you accountable. Since you are always responsible, it gets difficult to cheat on the things you planned to do because you made a clear commitment. When you train repeatedly, it becomes part of you. You can use a plan designed by this book, with just a few adjustments to suits your needs.

- **It provides structure:** You might start to feel your sessions are a waste of time. A workout plan gives you structure so that you don't get lost on what action to take next. You will always know what to do at every point in your mission.

- **It helps with consistency:** There won't always be time to fit in a workout. A workout plan will let you make your training a priority and be consistent with it through repetition. Your mind and body will learn to get accustomed to your new routine.

- **It provides and breaks down goals:** A workout plan gives you an automatic goal to complete the workout. You can easily break it down into tiny, achievable steps. Achieving every step serves as motivation to reach the next, and so on. You won't lose track of the successive line of action.

- **It helps prevent under or over training:** This is one of the most important reasons you should have a workout plan. Many people without a plan tend to either train too hard and put unnecessary stress on their bodies. You may be doing too much of a particular exercise. But when you have a plan, you won't suffer from a burnout. A good plan will give you a balance between workouts and rest. You may feel tired, or something might get in the way (as life tends to do); a schedule will allow you to see what you need to do and plan around life. There are so many factors that can go into under or over training.

- **It provides a record/checklist:** Your workout plan may include a log where you check off an achievement. This won't only serve as motivation but also evaluate the effectiveness of a particular workout program or specific programs. You can enhance your achievements and eliminate ineffective workout routines. Keeping track of your workouts also lets you know what's working and what could be changed. It's easier to share the experience with others when you have records.

For routine exercises, you can have the following workout exercises. Make sure to do them with perfect form and complete the prescribed sets and reps to the best of your ability. They've been handpicked just for men of your age.

- What is a rep? For any of you that are unaware, a repetition (rep) is one completed exercise movement –

from starting position to action and back to starting position.

- What is a set? A set is a certain number of reps. For instance, 8 to 12 reps can make up 1 set.

The main focus of this chapter is to give you a routine that you can use again and again for as long as you want. It should satisfy your fitness needs and get you on track to achieving the ideal physique for your age. Building muscle is never easy, no matter who you are. But if you follow my teachings to the best of your ability, you will possess the ticket that goes straight to the top.

This workout plan is crafted for maximum muscle growth, so I have incorporated gym equipment to achieve this. You may be getting angry while reading this now because I devoted a whole chapter to people without gym equipment, and now it seems like I am saying you need them. Please allow me to explain before writing a disgruntled review of this book. As stated before, I have chosen the exercises that I believe are the best for men over 50. Some are bodyweight exercises, and some require equipment. However, I understand that people have different circumstances, and you might not like what I have chosen for one reason or another.

To reconcile for this (before we get to the good stuff), I have made a shortlist of all the exercises mentioned in this book, along with the muscle group they belong to. This way, you can decide what to swap out without worrying about choosing the wrong exercise. Genius, I know. I got the idea from when I was a kid; I would go to the store and pick out five different candies, knowing they all tasted delicious. All I had to do was pick the ones I fancied that day. Here is the list. Enjoy.

Legs

Bodyweight:

- #1 The squat - glutes, hip flexors, and quadriceps
- #2 The lunge - hips, quads, glutes, hamstrings
- #3 The glute bridge - hamstrings and glutes
- #4 The fire hydrant - primarily glutes
- #5 The step-up - quads, glutes, hamstrings
- #6 The calf raise - primarily calf's

Dumbbell and resistance bands:

- #1 The dumbbell goblet squat - glutes, hip flexors, and quadriceps
- #2 The lunge with dumbbells - hips, quads, glutes, hamstrings
- #3 The resistance band squat - glutes, hip flexors, and quadriceps

Core - Abdomen

Bodyweight:

- #7 The crunch - upper and lower abdominal, oblique, and lower back
- #8 The flutter kick - lower abdominal and hip flexors
- #9 The Russian twist - all the abdominals and the oblique
- #12 The plank row - middle and upper back, core, shoulders, and arms
- #14 The Star plank - all the abdominals and the oblique
- # 15 The reach under plank - all the abdominals and the oblique

Dumbbell and resistance bands:

- #11 the dumbbell Russian twist - all the abdominals and the oblique
- #19 The Russian twist with resistance band - all the abdominals and the oblique
- #21 The woodchopper with resistance band - primarily oblique
- #22 The reverse crunch with resistance band - lower abdominals and obliques

Back

Bodyweight:

- #10 The superman - lower, upper back, and spinal muscles
- #11 The reverse snow angel - trapezius and lower back
- #12 The plank row - middle and upper back, core, shoulders, and arms

Dumbbell and resistance bands:

- #4 The bent-over dumbbell row - upper, mid, and lower back
- #10 The one-arm dumbbell row - lats and traps
- #16 The resistance band bent over row - middle and lower back
- #17 resistance band seated row - upper back

Chest

Bodyweight:

- #15 The push-up - pectorals, deltoids, and triceps
- The incline push-up - primarily pectorals
- The decline push-up - primarily upper pectorals
- The wide push-up - pectorals, deltoids, and triceps
- The incline push-up - pectorals, deltoids, and triceps

Dumbbell and resistance bands:

- #3 The dumbbell bench press - shoulders, triceps, forearms, lats, pectorals, and traps
- #18 The resistance band push-up - pectorals, deltoids, and triceps
- #23 The resistance band chest press - shoulders, triceps, forearms, lats, pectorals, and traps

Biceps

Bodyweight:

- #18 The side-lying bicep curl
- #19 The leg barbell curl

Dumbbell and resistance bands:

- #5 The dumbbell bicep curl
- #6 The cross-body dumbbell hammer curl
- #13 resistance band bicep curl

Triceps

Bodyweight:

- #20 The cobra push-up
- #21 The bodyweight tricep extension

Dumbbell and resistance bands:

#9 The overhead dumbbell tricep extension

#14 The resistance band overhead tricep extension

Shoulders - Deltoids

Bodyweight:

There aren't any good bodyweight exercises that isolate the shoulder, but all press-ups I've discussed work the shoulder muscles (deltoids), along with other muscle groups.

Dumbbell and resistance bands:

- #7 The dumbbell side lateral raise
- #8 The dumbbell shoulder press
- #15 The resistance band pull-apart
- #20 The resistance band overhead press

As you progress through the 4-week workout plan, you can swap any of the exercises with the ones mentioned above as long as they are in the same category, i.e., chest or legs.

A 4-WEEK WORKOUT PLAN

WEEK 1

Day 1:

2 - 3 minutes rest between each exercise.

- Lunge: 2 sets of 10 reps of each side with a 10-second gap between sets.
- Dumbbell Goblet Squat: 2 sets of 10 reps with a 10-second gap between sets
- Step Up: 2 sets of 10 reps of each side with a 10-second gap between sets.

Repeat the circuit once.

Day 2:

2 - 3 minutes rest between each exercise.

- Leg Barbell Curl: 2 sets of 15 reps of each side with a 10-second gap between sets.
- Plank row: 2 sets of 15 reps of each side with a 10-second gap between sets.
- Dumbbell Bicep Curl: 2 sets of 10 reps with a 10-second gap between sets.

Repeat the circuit once.

Day 3:

2 - 3 minutes rest between each exercise.

- Dumbbell Russian Twist: 3 sets of 8 – 12 reps, take 15 seconds before repeating set.
- Crunch: 3 sets of 10 – 15 reps with a 10-second gap

between sets.

Repeat the circuit once.

WEEK 2

Day 1:

2 minutes rest between each exercise.

- Reversed Snow Angel: 2 sets of 10 – 15 reps, with a 10-second gap between sets
- Resistance Band Pull Apart: 2 sets of 15 – 20 reps, with a 5-second gap between sets.
- Superman: Hold this position for 5 seconds and rest for 5 seconds, do 6 sets

Repeat the circuit one or two times.

Day 2:

2 minutes rest between each exercise.

- Calf Raise: 2 sets of 20 reps, with a 5-second gap between reps.
- Step Up: 2 sets of 10 reps of each side with a 10-second gap between sets.
- Resistance Band Squat: 2 sets of 10 reps with a 10-second gap between sets.

Repeat the circuit one or two times.

Day 3:

2 - 3 minutes rest between each exercise.

- Push-up: 2 sets of 10 – 15 reps with a 10-second gap between sets.
- Reach Under Plank: 2 sets of 10 – 15 reps with a 10-second gap between sets.

Repeat the circuit one or two times.

WEEK 3

Day 1: 3 minutes rest between each exercise.

- Resistance Band Bicep Curl: 2 sets of 8 – 12 reps with a 10-second gap between sets.
- Bodyweight Triceps Extension: 2 sets of 8 – 12 reps with a 10-second gap between sets.
- Cross-body Dumbbell Hammer Curl: 2 sets of 10 reps of each side with a 10-second gap between sets.

Repeat the circuit two to three times.

Day 2:

2 minutes rest between each exercise.

- Plank: Hold the plank position for 15 seconds, rest for 10 seconds, repeat three more times.
- Flutter Kick: Kick for 10 secs, rest and kick again, repeat three more times.
- Pilates Toe Tap: 2 sets of 10 reps of each side with a 10-second gap between sets.

Repeat the circuit two to three times.

Day 3:

2 minutes rest between each exercise.

- Quadruped Dumbbell Row: 3 sets of 8 – 12 reps of each side with a 10-second gap between sets.
- Wide Dumbbell Row: 3 sets of 8 – 12 reps of each side with a 10-second gap between sets.

Repeat the circuit two to three times.

WEEK 4

Day 1: 2 minutes rest between each exercise.

- Dumbbell Goblet Squat: 2 sets of 10 reps of each side with a 10-second gap between sets.
- Glute Bridge: 2 sets of 10 – 15 reps with a 10-second gap between sets.

- Fire Hydrant: 2 sets of 10 reps of each side with a 10-second gap between sets.

Repeat the circuit three to four times.

Day 2:

2 - 3 minutes rest between each exercise.

- Resistance Band Push-up: 3 sets of 10 reps with a 10-second gap between sets.
- Star Plank: Hold position for 5 seconds, return to starting position, rest, and hold the position again. Repeat for six times.

Repeat the circuit three to four times.

Day 3:

2 - 3 minutes rest between each exercise.

- Dumbbell Side Lateral Raise: 2 sets of 10 reps with a 10-second gap between sets.
- Side-Lying Bicep Curl: 2 sets of 5 reps of each side with a 10-second gap between sets.
- Overhead Dumbbell Press: 8 reps of a single set. Be sure to use lightweight dumbbells.

Repeat the circuit three to four times.

TIPS FOR YOUR WORKOUTS.

Warm-up first: This helps prepare your body. It gradually increases your cardiovascular system by raising your temperature and allowing more blood flow to your muscles. It may also reduce soreness and your risk of injury. You can warm up with any of these exercises: knee to chest, quad stretch, lunge with overhead reach, and rotation or wide stance shift. A 5-minute warm-up is all you need, so try not to focus on this too much.

Workout Schedule: A scheduled workout is a scheduled appointment. When you plan your workouts, you develop a balance of strength, flexibility, and cardio training every week. If you lack consistency, you may be tempted to fall back on something relatively easy and quick so that you can fit in on that particular day or time. So you must schedule the days of the week you'll be exercising and stay true to it.

You should work out three times a week or two if you're feeling a lot of fatigue. But always take the next day after a workout to rest. That is when your muscles go into recovery mode; exercising while in this state would not provide a lot of muscle growth and could lead to injures. The same principles apply with exercising the same muscle groups back to back; even if you have a rest day in between, muscle fatigue increases. In every sense, it is wise to work all of the muscle groups one after the other during the week. Lastly, choose a specific time for a workout, either early in the morning or late in the evening, whatever suits your needs. However, once you have selected a time, try to stay loyal to it; it will help you develop a long-lasting exercise habit.

This routine is manufactured to push you every week, but you must understand that everyone is different. You might find that as you advance through the weeks, you start to notice that the activities have become underwhelming, or maybe they were too easy in the first place. On the other hand, you might find that you're frequently struggling to finish all of the sets, and your body aches too much the next day. Although we all share something in common, everyone is reading this book with slightly different circumstances. Our growth varies from person to person.

If either of these apply to you, I urge you to use some initiative and listen to your body. Feeling soreness the day after a workout is usual, but if it's stopping you from engaging in your daily activities, you should alter the plan. Keep the same level of consistency but take a couple of reps off the next time.

Conversely, the same can be said when the workout plan gets too easy. Don't use this time to relax; instead, pick up the pace, so you feel that burn again. The holy grail of muscle building is progressive overloading. Meaning once you reach a level of muscle strength, you have to increase the difficulty to hit the level above that, and so o

6

THE SIXTH KEY

THE ULTIMATE DUO: DIET AND EXERCISE

A couple of days ago, I watched a game of soccer with my friends, and I heard the commentator remark, *"you can't keep scoring own goals and expect to win the match."* You can perceive this as a metaphor for your training. You can't keep tearing down what you are building and expect it to stand. A body divided against itself is a week body.

People often wish to live healthily and stay fit, they start many healthy practices to achieve their goals, but unfortunately, they hold on to unhealthy tendencies that draw them back three steps for every two steps they gain. If you acquire one bad habit to lose another, have you even made any changes?

It's a commended step you've taken to train after 50. However, you need more than training to live that healthy and fit lifestyle; you need the proper diet. At this age, you cannot continue to get away with the bad eating habits you had in your younger years. For example, you could consume many calories as a young man in your 30s and still not have issues with excessive weight, but you cannot afford to do that now. Your immune system is not as durable as it used to be. You need to cover all bases when staying healthy and fit at this age. The proper nutrients are the key to this, and I will walk you through it.

Let's discuss the nutrients you need at this age.

FOOD FOR THOUGHT

Your body needs nutrients to stay active and grow; however, some nutrients will do your body more good at this stage in your life than others. Let's take a look at some of the nutrients you need.

Calcium and Vitamin D

Calcium and vitamin D supplements reduce the risk of falling in older adults by improving muscle strength, muscle function, balance and reducing bone loss. Increasing food intake will enhance your muscle growth; it's a step in the right direction.

Older men need more calcium and vitamin D to help them maintain strong and healthy bones. Foods that are rich in calcium include:

- Low-fat and free fat dairy products, like milk and yogurt.
- Fortified foods and beverages, such as some cereals.

Dark green leafy vegetables and canned fish are also sources of calcium. Fatty fish like salmon, eggs, and fortified foods and beverages are rich in vitamin D. It is advisable to have three servings of low-fat and free fat every day. If you take calcium supplements, then make sure to choose one with vitamin D.

Dietary Fiber

Fiber helps you maintain a normal bowel function and improve digestive health by the survival of good bacteria. Studies have shown that when you take more dietary fiber, it helps reduce the risk of developing Type 2 diabetes and heart disease. Since foods rich in fiber take longer to digest, they can help you stay full longer, so you don't get the temptation to snack. As a man over 50 years, you need at least 30 grams of dietary fiber every day. Whole grains, beans, fruits, vegetables, and lentils are good sources of fiber. Try making at least half of your grain intake whole grain. Good whole grain sources are pasta, oatmeal, whole-wheat bread, and whole-grain cereals. If you're buying processed fiber food, make sure to check the label for nutritional facts, ensure it has at least 3 grams of dietary fiber per serving.

Vitamin B12

Vitamin B12, also known as cobalamin, is an essential vitamin and is not produced in the body. It can only be obtained from food or supplements. The recommended daily intake for you is 2.4mcg (micrograms). Vitamin B helps with red blood cell formation, preventing anemia, supporting bone health, and preventing osteoporosis. If you combine this with your strength training, you will be well on your way to achieving strong, healthy bones. It can also reduce an eye disease that mainly affects your central vision, called macular degeneration, a disease often associated with advancement in age.

Potassium

Potassium is one of the major macro minerals. It plays a massive role in the function of the kidneys, heart, muscles, and transmission of messages through the nervous system. As a man over 50 years, you need about 3500mg consumption of potassium per day. Good sources of potassium include fruits and vegetables, such as bananas, sweet potatoes, spinach, and white beans.

Another benefit of taking potassium is it helps to prevent or manage high blood pressure and cardiovascular diseases. It also plays a role in bone health. Studies have shown that those who take lots of fruits and vegetables containing potassium may have higher bone mineral density. A diet that's high in potassium may also help preserve muscle mass in older people.

Healthy Fats

At this age, most of the fats you should eat now should come from heart-healthy monounsaturated and polyunsaturated fats, found in fish, nuts, vegetable oils, avocados, and seeds. Saturated fats, which come from fatty meat and full-fat dairy, should be limited to help reduce the risk of heart disease.

Zinc

Zinc is an essential mineral. If your zinc levels are low, testosterone and insulin sensitivity can dip. (Fun fact), it also plays a role in reducing the duration of the common cold. We lose zinc through sweat, so it's vital to keep an adequate intake. Food sources are lean meat, shellfish, legumes, seeds, nuts, eggs, whole grains, etc.

Omega-3 Fish Oil (EPA/DHA)

Omega-3 fatty acids are a class of polyunsaturated fatty acids. Three main types are essential within this class: DHA, EPA, and ALA. It's imperative to consume EPA and DHA in your diet because your body can synthesize them. Fish is the primary food source, but if you can't eat fish up to three times every week, you can get the nutrients needed in supplements. Fish oils benefit your health in many ways: they boost heart health by negating risk factors for heart disease like high cholesterol, triglyceride levels, and blood pressure. Additionally, they fight long-term inflammation and promote proper inflammatory responses and recovery. Finally, they help with joint health by improving the body's range of motion and reducing morning stiffness.

Probiotics

Probiotics are living microorganisms that have health benefits when consumed. There are billions of living bacteria in our body that make up what we call the microbiome. There are good bacteria and bad ones that have several functions and effects on our health. Our microbiome changes from time to time and is unique to each individual based on how we relate to our environment, consume medication, and many other factors. With its effect on our body, consuming probiotic supplements regularly is very helpful to maintaining your microbiome.

Curcumin

Curcumin is the most powerful naturally occurring anti-inflammatory ingredient found in turmeric. Curcumin can help combat chronic inflammation that can be disruptive to healthy cellular processes.

Electrolytes

They are a group of minerals in our body with an electric charge. Hence the name. They have many functions that help to maintain homeostasis. Two of these include regulating fluid balance and muscle contractions. This is why it's among the best supplements for men who work out. Our kidneys do substantial work in maintaining fluid balance, and if we take appropriate and healthy diets, electrolyte supplements might not be needed.

Make Calories Count

You cannot eat the same way you did in your 20s and 30s while maintaining a healthy weight. Those days you burned more calories because your body was more active, but now, you don't naturally burn as much. Your metabolism has slowed down, and you'll need more activity to keep it up.

Despite the fact you need fewer calories, you need the same or possibly higher amounts of nutrients as you grow older. Ensure you include wholesome foods regularly, including fruits, vegetables, low-fat or fat-free dairy, whole grains, lean proteins, and healthy plant-based fats, which will give you nutrients and help keep those calories in check.

Note: Nutrients that might not be readily available in food should be taken in supplements.

As I quoted at the beginning of this chapter, "you can't keep scoring own goals and expect to win the match." We have discussed the nutrients you need at this age. However, there are some things you need to avoid as well. Let's take a look at them:

Sodium

You don't generally need to look for sodium because it will always find you. The key is avoiding it. Almost any unprocessed food like fruits, whole grain, nuts, vegetables, meat, and dairy foods is low in sodium. And most of the salt in our diets is from foods commercially prepared. Notable sources of sodium in our diets include breads/rolls, savory snacks (chips, popcorn, pretzels, crackers), sandwiches, cold cuts/cured meats, soups, pizza, burritos, tacos, chicken, cheese, eggs, omelets. Unfortunately, these are foods most of us don't want to do without.

Salt, also known as sodium chloride, is roughly 60% chloride and 40% sodium. It's used to flavor food along with other things. It's also used as a food preservative because bacteria can't live in the presence of high amounts of salt. Although, the human body requires a small amount of sodium to contract and relax muscles, carry out nerve impulses, and maintain the proper balance of water and minerals. An estimated 500mg of sodium is needed for these vital functions every day. Too much sodium in your diet can then lead to high blood pressure, heart disease, and possibly even a stroke. It can also cause a loss of calcium. If you consume a teaspoon of salt every day, that's about 2300mg of sodium, which is way far above what your body needs.

In many people, the kidneys have trouble keeping up with excess sodium in the blood. As sodium accumulates, the body needs water to dilute the sodium. This will cause an increase in the fluid surrounding the cells and the amount of blood in the bloodstream. When blood increases, the heart has to do more work, and there is more pressure on blood vessels, which leads to high blood pressure, heart attack, and stroke. You're also at risk of heart failure. These are extreme cases, so please refrain from throwing your salt shaker in the trash. Evidence has shown that too much salt can damage the aorta, heart, and kidneys, even without an increase in blood pressure, and it may be bad for the bones too.

Since salt tends to be a flavor we long for, here are some alternatives to flavoring your foods while avoiding too much salt intake: dill, cinnamon, basil, nutmeg, and rosemary. These are all very low in sodium.

Saturated fats

We are surrounded by lots of this, though, not like sodium. Saturated fat is a type of dietary fat found in animals mostly; some plants also contain them. Saturated fats are without a doubt unhealthy for you. Foods such as butter, red meat, palm oil, palm kernel oil, coconut oil, and cheese contain high concentrations of saturated fats.

Your body needs healthy fats for fuel and many other functions. Too much saturated fats can cause cholesterol to build up in your blood vessels. Saturated fat increases your LDL (bad) cholesterol. And high LDL cholesterol will increase your chances of heart disease and strokes. Many high-fat foods such as baked foods, fried foods have lots of saturated fats. Overeating it can add extra calories to your diet and cause you to add excessive weight, and I'm sure you don't want to add that excess weight at this time.

Processed Foods

Processed foods have been altered during preparation to make them more tasteful, flavorful, convenient, or improve shelf life. Some foods are more processed than others. For example, a box of macaroni and cheese is considered heavily processed because it's chemically altered with artificial flavors, additives, and other ingredients. Most of the foods we eat have been processed to a lesser degree, but the immediate concern here is about ultra-processed foods such as cake mixes, jarred pasta sauces, crackers, and many more.

There are lots of potential health risks in consuming ultra-processed foods. So much processing deprives foods of their nutrients, which means you'll only be consuming and not getting the expected benefits because the nutrients are stripped away in the process. You stand the temptation of overeating if you frequently indulge in processed foods. This will always put you above your maximum calorie intake for a day. And what is worse – most ultra-processed foods are calorie-dense and are pretty addictive. Also, most processed foods digest quicker, and we burn about half as many calories digesting processed foods compared to unprocessed foods – if you combine this with the fact that these foods are calorie-dense, then it's a straight road to weight gain. These foods are also filled with many artificial ingredients, most have not been tested by any other person other than the company using them, and these ingredients might be unsafe for your health. More so, too much processed food may result in obesity, heart disease, high blood pressure, and diabetes because most of these foods contain too much sugar, sodium, and fat.

I realize it will be tough to do without processed foods 100% of the time, but you should understand it is a process, and progress is more important than perfection. Always check the label; a general rule of thumb is the longer the ingredient list, the more processed the food is. And if you can't pronounce most of the ingredients, that's a hint that the food is ultra-processed. Start replacing them slowly, start by cooking more meals when you are at home. Everyone has to start somewhere.

Lower Calories

The amount of calories you need per day depends on your age and activity level. The daily calories you need over 50 are approximately:

2,000 to 2,200 calories if you are not active.

2,200 to 2,400 calories if you are moderately active.

2,400 to 2,800 calories if you are regularly active.

You might be wondering why you should avoid lower calories when earlier on, you were advised against higher calories – balance is the key; not too much, not too little. Just as eating more than your body needs causes you to gain weight, eating fewer than your body needs causes you to lose weight. Some effects of lower calories include:

It can lower your metabolism: Eating fewer calories than your body needs can cause your metabolism to slow down. And more than that, a slow metabolism can continue even after a person increases their calory intake. Another way lower calories can affect your body is muscle loss, especially if your diet is low in protein and you fail to include any exercise in your life.

It can cause fatigue and nutrient deficiency: You stand the risk of getting fatigued frequently and facing challenges in meeting your daily nutrient needs. There is a lot of chance you're not taking sufficient amounts of some nutrients if your calorie intake is lower than it should be. For instance, insufficient amounts of iron, folate, or vitamin B12 can lead to anemia. An inadequate amount of protein intake can lead to muscle loss. An Insufficient amount of vitamin A can weaken your immune system and lead to permanent eye damage. The list goes on.

It can weaken your bones: Lower calorie intake can weaken your bones. This is because lower calories reduce hormone levels like testosterone and estrogen. Low levels of these hormones can cause a reduction in bone formation and increase bone breakdown, which results in weaker bones. Also, if you combine lower calorie intake with physical exercises, it can increase stress hormone levels, leading to bone loss. Bone loss is no joke; it's irreversible and increases the risk of fractures.

It may lower your immunity: You are at risk of infections and illnesses when you drop your calorie intake, and of course, this is not good for you. A study comparing athletes in sports focused on cutting weight, such as boxing, to those in sports less focused on body weight. The researchers found out that athletes in fields focused on weight control made more were almost twice as likely to become ill in the study period of three months.

Change is one of the hardest things we often face. Even though there are many benefits to changing a lifestyle, we find it difficult to do. It's because change threatens us; puts more pressure on us; takes us out of our comfort zones; requires more than what we are used to. But it is something we must address. And not just change in any direction but in the right direction. Because without change, we won't grow; in fact, we can't grow.

I understand how difficult it will be to do without processed foods – the pizzas, cakes, cookies, and many more. That will mean being extra conscious of what you eat, especially anytime you are not home. It can be tedious trying to fill in the vitamins, calcium, magnesium into one's daily meal, regardless of appetite for these foods or not. But these are sacrifices one must make - the ones who do reek the rewards.

The key to making this change without much inconvenience is doing it slowly. Many people try to stop a habit or an addiction abruptly, but only for a short time, and before long, they're back. So, take it slowly. You're not in a competition. It's OK to plan how you want to include the nutrients you need into your daily meal and how you want to avoid the things you don't need. Slowly drop the negatives and add the positives. I bet you, before long, it becomes part of you.

Take your nutrition with as much care as you can muster. It's crucial to your strength training goals, and more so, to your overall well-being.

7

THE SEVENTH KEY

A SHIELD FOR STRENGTH TRAINING

Many people start training, injure themselves, and never train again. As I've said earlier, the goal is to train and build muscle, not sustain injury. So, make safety a priority.

There is a common mistake with many of us – we want something, and we want it so bad that we disregard the aspects that don't get us there as quickly as possible. You cannot cut corners with strength training. Any attempt to do so will result in a high risk of long-lasting injuries.

You want to be fit, build muscle mass, lose weight, and many more. I am sure you understand but let me reiterate that you cannot accomplish these wonderful aspirations in a day, week, or month. It takes a lot of time and patience, just like anything worth having in life. Please refrain from operating weights you know are too heavy, and try not to push your body too far. You only get one, and it should be treated with the utmost care. Follow the plan mapped out for you in chapter six. And with time, you'll see the results of your labor.

Safety First

I don't think there's anyone aged 50 who wouldn't have come across the phrase, "safety first." It's a common saying. But what does it mean? It means before all things, there must be a condition whereby you're protected from the situation that could likely cause you harm. That's what we're going to cover in the final chapter of your training.

Visit your doctor: This should be the first thing you do, see your doctor before starting an exercise program. Especially if you're overweight, you have a pre-existing health condition, or haven't exercised before. The pre-exercise screening will inform your doctor of health conditions that may put you at greater risk, which may outweigh the potential benefits of exercising. It is a deeply bitter pill to swallow but a super necessary one if it could cause you harm.

Always warm-up before any physical exercise: We touched on this earlier in the book but let me further explain. Suppose you're a beginner who hasn't had any experience working out before. In that case, I'll advise you to take two days to perform some aerobic exercises: 30 minutes each day of either walking, swimming or riding a bicycle. This will help prepare your muscles for the stress you're going to put them under. Furthermore, before starting each session (regardless of experience), you need a 5 minute warm-up of walking or any other light aerobic exercise.

Safety tips for strength training: If you consult with your doctor, they will inform you of any precautions you should take, but in case they don't, here are some suggestions for staying safe.

- Carry out exercises using the proper technique. If you're unsure how to do an exercise correctly, you should ask a fitness coach, gym instructor, or strength training physiologist for help.
- Start slowly. I've spoken about this before. If you're just starting out, you may find you can only lift just a few kilograms; it's fine. Once your muscles are getting the required strength from the repetition of training, you'll be surprised at the rate of progression. Once you can do 12 to 15 reps with a particular weight, gradually increase the weight or the reps.
- Never use faulty equipment to train. You'll increase your risk of injury that way. Use only safe and well-managed equipment. We don't want you dropping a weight on your foot from using a dodgy dumbbell.
- Don't halt your breath while training. Breathe at a consistent level when you're lifting by breathing out during the exertion and breathing in during the

relaxation. This is how I do it, but if it's more comfortable to do it the other way, that's perfectly acceptable.

- Be in control of the weights at all times. Please do not throw them up or down or use momentum in swinging the weight through the range of motion. Aside from the injuries you could sustain, it is not an effective way to train.

Maintain a strong positioning when you're lifting. It will prevent injury.

- Lift weights you know you can. Stop if you feel the weight is too heavy to control. It never hurts to test the amount of weight by picking it up first.
- Use the full range of motion. It is imperative when you're lifting a weight that you let it travel through the full range of motion of the joint. This will develop the strength of your muscles and balance out the load to increase stability and overall movement. It will also decrease your chances of injury through overstretching.
- Wear clothes appropriate for a workout and safety equipment like gloves. You should wear comfortable clothes that don't restrict movement and allow you to sweat freely.
- Maintain correct posture and body position at all

times. Practice actively posturing yourself while walking or sitting to help you get used to it.

- When you complete a set, place the weight on the floor gently, don't drop them. If not, you could injure yourself or someone around you. I am guilty of this sometimes, and it has ended in me effing and blinding at a sore toe.

- Don't train if you're too tired or feeling sick. It's not worth it, and your body needs to focus on recovery.

- Don't train if you're injured. Stop your exercise at once and seek medical care.

- Muscles need time to repair and grow after they've been worked. You should always rest your muscles for at least 24 hours before training the same muscle group again.

Safety is paramount. So it would be best if you didn't take those safety tips for granted. Given that, I'll be giving you four more workout exercises that are very safe for training lower back pain and strengthening your back. I frequently suffer from back pain, so I know how painful it can be, but these exercises are an excellent natural remedy for the pain. I hope they help.

1. CAT COW

A gentle flow between two poses warms your body and brings flexibility to your spine. It stretches your back and neck, softly stimulating and strengthening your abdominal organs. Cat cow also opens your chest, encouraging slow, deep breathing. Your kidneys and adrenal glands get stimulated by the spinal movement of the two poses. Coordinating these moves with your breath relieves you of stress and calms your mind. You are also helping to develop postural awareness and balance throughout your body. It brings your spine into correct alignment and can help you ease back pain when you practice it regularly.

How to exercise:

- Start on all four on your hands and knees, as in a crawling position. Ensure you keep your wrists are directly below your shoulders and knees directly under the hips. Your fingertips pointing straight in front of you, and your shins and knees kept at hip-width apart. Begin with your head in a neutral position, looking downward.
- Begin by moving into a cow pose; that being, you slowly curve your spine inward and drop your stomach down, taking a deep breath in as you do so and aim your head up to the sky.
- Next, move into the cat pose, reverse the position of your spine in one smooth transition so that you end with your spine curved upward, pointing to the ceiling. Breathe out as you do this and point your head down into your body. That's a rep.

You can do 15 reps of the cat-cow, rest a while and have another set.

2. HOLLOW BODY CRUNCH

It's an intermediate to advanced level abdominal exercise that targets your core muscles. It's an excellent move for targeting the transverse abdominis, obliques, hip flexors, quads, rectus abdominis, erector spinae, and inner thighs. When done correctly, the hollow body crunch can improve your posture. Also, if the lower back and abs are in the correct position, this move will help with strengthening the muscles needed to prevent lower back pain.

How to exercise:

- Start by lying on your exercise mat, your legs and arms extended with your body going in a straight line from fingertips to your toes. Then, raise both arms and legs about 6 inches above the ground.
- Make sure to contract your abs by engaging your core.
- Move your arms and legs to meet until the elbow touches the knees, then return to starting position. That is a rep.

You can do ten reps, rest a while, then have another set or move onto something else.

3. QUADRUPED OPPOSITE ARM-LEG RAISE

The quadruped opposite arm-leg raise exercise, commonly referred to as bird-dog, strengthens your lower back. It primarily targets the erector spinal muscles, which run along your spine and are in charge of extending your torso. If you want to develop strength in your lower back to reduce the risk of injury due to muscular weakness, this exercise is the one for you.

How to exercise:

- As in a crawling position, you start on all four - your hands directly under your shoulders and knees directly under your hips. Your spine should be neutral throughout the moves.
- Extend your left arm forward while at the same time, you extend your right leg up and backward until both limbs are parallel to the floor.
- Hold that position for a few seconds, then return to starting position. Repeat for the other sides.

4. KNEE TO CHEST STRETCH

It is used to stretch your lower back and hip muscles. It also helps relieve pressure on spinal nerves by creating more space for them as they exit the spine. I advise you utilize this stretch after every workout.

How to exercise:

- Lie on your back. Bend your knees and glue your feet flat on the floor.
- Bring one of your knees to your chest while keeping the other leg on the floor. Ensure you keep your lower back pressed to the floor. Hold the position for about 15 to 30 seconds.
- Relax and return the knee to the starting pairing. Repeat the process for your other leg.
- To get more stretched, put out your other leg straight instead of bent at the knee while one is at your chest.

Exercises to avoid

Not all exercises are good, nor suitable for beginners. In fact, some could lead to injury in the process of training. It would be best if you stayed clear of them. I've carefully selected some exercises you should stay away from at 50 years+.

Bar Muscle-up: You should never try this exercise which involves hanging on a bar and swinging yourself up and down the bar. Pushing yourself up and down the bar is a challenging exercise, especially if you're overweight. It can only be an effective exercise if you are already good at performing them. Even so, they put a lot of stress on your shoulder joints and ligaments. At your age, they are not a worthy exercise; regular pull-ups can provide more muscle activation because you can perform more of them safely.

Upright Dip: This is a bit similar to the muscle-up. You push yourself up and down a very low bar. You can strain, wear and tear your arm doing this too. Plus, easing a grip on the bar will result in a fall which can be damaging.

Kipping Pull-up: They are a variation on the standard pull-up, which involves a swinging motion of the body, accompanied by a sudden burst of power from the shoulders to reach above the bar. This exercise is a high injury risk exercise, as your shoulders get violently pulled on every rep. And it's not as effective as a standard pull-up – the only reason it's used is for competition in sports like cross-fit, whereby you have to do as many pull-ups as quickly as possible. It is grossly inferior to the strict pull-up in terms of building strength.

Behind the Neck Pull-up: This is another dangerous exercise for you. Using any lat pull-down machine behind your head is bad for you. It forces you to extend your shoulders unnaturally. Even if you're super flexible, it still puts unneeded tension on your shoulder joints. It puts you at the risk of injuring your rotator cuffs. You are also prone to injuring yourself because you can't see the bar behind your head.

Back To the Wall Handstand Push-up: You start this exercise standing on your two hands, your legs leaning against the wall while your back faces the wall. This puts increased pressure on your arms because you are essentially stuck in this position with the weight of your body bearing down on the shoulders until you finish the set. It might result in strain, wear, or muscle tear of the arms. Lastly, if you do not have total control and your muscles get fatigued during your set, then it could result in your face smooshed against the floor. It would help if you stayed off this exercise.

Behind the Neck Press: It's a futile exercise for building the upper body strength because it can put a vast strain on your shoulder and neck muscles. Unfortunately, many people suffer from issues surrounding these areas of the body when you get older, such as rounded shoulders and lower back pain. It can commonly be attributed to the nature of their jobs if this applies to you. Behind the neck press should be a no-go zone.

Sit-up: Although it is widely practiced among fitness enthusiasts, you might be doing it at the expense of your spine's health. It can cause wear and tear of the spine through repetitive flexion, worsening your posture. Your abdominal core muscles should stabilize your spine, not encouraging flexion. And sit-ups can lead to lumbar spinal injury, predominantly if you previously suffered lower back pain. Lastly, they are not a functional movement of the body. Meaning you don't need sit-ups to improve any function or activity you do daily.

Pseudo Pull-Up: The pull-up and chin-up are both fantastic exercises. But if you're not doing the chin-up exercise correctly, you're probably doing a pseudo-pull-up. And pseudo-pull-ups only give reassurance that you're performing a full range of motion reps and can cause you neck pain.

Chair Dip: The chair dip variation of the dip exercise is an awful exercise because many people lack adequate shoulder range of motion to perform this movement safely and effectively. This exercise requires a great deal of shoulder extension you can't find in many people. It puts excessive wear on the shoulder joints from an extreme internal rotation. And it could worsen your posture by encouraging forward shoulder position.

Upright Row: You use two dumbbells or a barbell for this. You're required to position your shoulders into internal rotation with these weights. This puts your rotator cuff into a compromising posture and could lead to shoulder infringement, causing wear and tear on your rotator.

Behind The Neck Pulldown: This exercise is performed on a cable Lat Pull-down machine. Instead of pulling the weight down the chest, it is pulled down behind the neck. It leaves your neck in a cranked position and can strain the posterior neck muscles.

Loaded Back Hyper-Extensions: This exercise involves you getting on a back raise machine, holding a weight on your chest, and going to town bending at the spine down, and then all the way back up until you can't anymore. This causes far too much stress. Your low back should never be extended past its natural capabilities. Hyperextending the low back can lead to a disc injury.

Shrugs: This exercise is not particularly harmful, but many people perform it with too much weight and reps. Excessive weight often results in an improper position, leading to severe neck muscle strain. Feel free to perform this exercise but take caution with the weight you are using.

In closing this chapter, I want you to learn as many of these tips for staying as much as you possibly can. You may not notice the differences at first, but often when it comes to safety, if nothing goes wrong, it means you're doing it right. This book aims to create a long-lasting body for you that you can be confident in relying on.

CONCLUSION

The numerous benefits of strength training can never be overemphasized. It doesn't matter how old you are. You are never too late to the party. You should know the much-touted loss of muscle mass due to aging is even more so because of physical inactivity. Strength training can help you build that muscle mass, protect your bone health, regulate excess weight, manage chronic diseases, and many more. If you want to stay fit, strong, and healthy – strength training has got you covered. These are all things you should know and be an expert in by now if you have been following along.

The unknown is a scary thing. You might find the thought of making this kind of commitment intimidating as a beginner as it forces you to leave your warm comfort zone. The same can be said if you have experience in strength training but only stuck with the same routine. A transition to a new way of exercising puts you right back in that beginner stage. However, it would help if you didn't think of this as a bad thing. A fighter in the UFC once said, "I go into every training session a novice. If you surround yourself by lesser men that baby you, you gain nothing". Approaching your workouts with a beginner's mindset will open your mind and allow you to learn.

You only need to find the right motivation – top of which is the reason you decided to train. This will hold you up through thick and thin. Creating time for training might appear a Herculean task, but if you prioritize your time, you'll find yourself with an abundance of it.

Start your training slowly and steadily. Set goals as you start your program. If you have no purpose or destination in mind, you will most likely fail. Put effort into visualizing one. Be patient when you start. A bottle of fine wine takes years to mature. Exercise patience!

Although you do not need any equipment (as I have proven), that does not mean it's not a wise investment. And besides, it's fun buying new toys! There is very cheap equipment, from the resistance bands to medicine balls. You don't need to spend a lot on equipment at the start. With a pair of dumbbells and resistance bands, you'll have everything you need to make incredible gains without draining your pocket. You'll find it's worth your investment, and you'll be glad you did. Without any equipment at all, you can still achieve your strength training goal – all you need is the weight of your own body. Bodyweight workouts have been proven efficient and effective for strength training. And, as a beginner over 50, I advise you to start with bodyweight workouts to help you gain some form before venturing into using weights. The last piece of advice I can give you on this topic is to save the gym machines for later on down the line. Get your body familiar with the consistent activities, and then move onto something more challenging. I will write another book covering this, so keep an eye out!

Have a workout plan – those who fail to plan, plan to fail. A workout plan has been designed to suit YOU. Ensure you give it a try for at least four weeks to get the full effects. It helps you stay on course and train effectively. Ensure you're consistent, and remember to progressively overload your muscles with more reps or higher weight.

Take care of your diet. This is very important. You can't afford to live a carefree or careless life in this regard. Your diets make or break your strength training workouts. There are nutrients beneficial to your body that you must prioritize. And if you can't get them sufficiently in foods, take them in supplements. On the other side, you need to avoid food that will worsen your health. One of them is processed foods. Ultra-processed foods are very detrimental to your health. Also, avoid taking lower calories. It mars your strength training amidst other harmful effects.

Lastly, you need to stay safe. The goal is to sustain fitness, muscle mass, etc., not sustain injuries - exercise properly. Don't rush through. Don't attempt weights that are too heavy for you. Some workout exercises are too strenuous for you as a beginner; some are strenuous because you're of age, don't attempt these exercises. I've listed them out for you, so you shouldn't have any problems. And as I advised, if you feel it's unsafe for you, stay clear of it. There are hundreds of other safe exercises for you. Your safety matters so much.

Now that you've been fully prepared go out and build that strong, fit and healthy body. The most important thing in your training is to have fun and be happy doing the things you love. Hopefully, strength training can become one of those things on your list of happiness. Just like it is on mine.

If you found enjoyment reading this book or learned something from it, I kindly ask that you leave me a review. It shows me that people care. Thank you until the next time and good luck!

REFERENCES

Academy of Nutrition and Dietetics, 2020. Nutrition for older men https://www.eatright.org/health/wellness/healthy-aging/nutrition-for-older-men#:~:text=Men%20older%20than%2050%20need,can%20all%20be%20good%20sources

Alina Petre, 2017. 5 Ways Restricting Calories Can Be Harmful. https://www.healthline.com/nutrition/calorie-restriction-risks#TOC_TITLE_HDR_7

America Heart Association, 2018. Strength and Resistance Training Exercise https://www.heart.org/en/healthy-living/fitness/fitness-basics/strength-and-resistance-training-exercise

Casino.org, 2020. 10 Boxers Who Started Late https://www.-google.com/amp/s/www.casino.org/blog/10-boxers-who-started-late/amp/

Chris Iliades, 2019. 7 Ways Strength Training Boosts Your Health and Fitness. https://www.everydayhealth.com/fitness/add-strength-training-to-your-workout.aspx

Jeanne Bellezzo, 2018. Is Comparing Sabotaging Your Success? https://www.acefitness.org/education-and-resources/lifestyle/blog/7021/is-comparison-sabotaging-your-success/

John C. Maxwell, 2002. Leadership 101

Justin C. Strickland and Mark A. Smith, 2014. The anxiolytic effects of resistance exercise

K. Aleisha Fetters, 2018. 11 Benefits of Strength Training That Have Nothing to Do With Muscle Size https://health.usnews.com/wellness/fitness/articles/2018-03-23/11-benefits-of-strength-training-that-have-nothing-to-do-with-muscle-size

Kaitlyn Berkheiser, 2018. 9 Health Benefits of Vitamin B12, Based on Science

https://www.healthline.com/nutrition/vitamin-b12-benefits#TOC_TITLE_HDR_4

Kristen M Beavers et al, 2017. Effect of Exercise Type During Intentional Weight Loss on Body Composition in Older Adults with Obesity

Megan Ware, 2021. Everything you need to know about potassium https://www.medicalnewstoday.com/articles/287212#recommended-intake

Robert J. Davis, 2018. 7 Simple Ways To Motivate Yourself To Exercise. https://www.google.com/amp/s/time.com/5105991/how-to-build-self-discipline-to-exercise/%3famp=true

Steven L Watson Benjamin K Weeks Lisa J Weis Amy T Harding Sean A Horan Belinda R Beck, 2017. High-Intensity Resistance and Impact Training Improves Bone Mineral Density and Physical Function in Postmenopausal Women With Osteopenia and Osteoporosis: The LIFTMOR Randomized Controlled Trial https://asbmr.onlinelibrary.wiley.com/doi/full/10.1002/jbmr.3284

U.S. Department of Health and Human Services, 2018. Physical Activity Guidelines for Americans

UW Health, Health and Wellness

https://www.uwhealth.org/health-wellness/what-you-need-to-know-about-low-t/51045

Withings, 2021. How Muscle Mass Shapes Your Health

https://www.withings.com/us/en/health-insights/about-muscle-mass-benefits#grow

Printed in Great Britain
by Amazon

64175596R00118